WORKBOOK FOR RADIATION PROTECTION

IN

MEDICAL RADIOGRAPHY

WORKBOOK FOR RADIATION PROTECTION

IN

MEDICAL RADIOGRAPHY

FIFTH EDITION

MARY ALICE STATKIEWICZ SHERER, AS, RT(R), FASRT

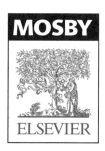

MOSBY

ELSEVIER

11830 Westline Industrial Drive
St. Louis, Missouri 63146

WORKBOOK FOR RADIATION PROTECTION IN MEDICAL
RADIOGRAPHY

ISBN-13: 978-0-323-04476-9
ISBN-10: 0-323-04476-X

ISBN-13: 978-0-323-04476-9
ISBN-10: 0-323-04476-X

Managing Editor: Mindy Hutchinson
Associate Developmental Editor: Christina Pryor
Publishing Services Manager: Julie Eddy
Project Manager: Rich Barber

Printed in the United States

Last digit is the print number: 9 8 7 6 5 4 3

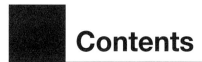

Contents

1 Introduction to Radiation Protection

Chapter 1 provides an introduction to radiation protection that includes discussion of the use of ionizing radiation in the healing arts, beginning with the discovery of x-rays in 1895. The following topics are covered in this chapter: effective radiation protection, biologic effects, justification and responsibility for radiologic procedures, diagnostic efficacy, occupational and nonoccupational dose limits, the as low as reasonably achievable (ALARA) principle, patient protection and patient education, risk versus potential benefit of radiologic procedures, and use of background equivalent radiation time (BERT) to inform patients of the amount of radiation they will receive during a specific x-ray procedure. The chapter also discusses types of radiation, the electromagnetic spectrum, particulate radiation, equivalent dose and effective dose, the biologic damage potential of ionizing radiation, natural and manmade sources of radiation, the accidents at the Three Mile Island-2 (TMI-2) and Chernobyl nuclear power plants, and the use of diagnostic x-ray machines and radiopharmaceuticals in medicine.

CHAPTER HIGHLIGHTS

- Ionizing radiation has both a beneficial and a destructive potential.
- Healthy, normal biologic tissue can be injured by ionizing radiation, therefore human beings must be protected against significant and continuous exposure.
- X-rays are a form of ionizing radiation, therefore their use in medicine to detect disease and injury requires protective measures.
- Effective radiation protection measures should always be used when diagnostic imaging procedures are performed in order to safeguard patients, personnel, and the general public.
- Radiation exposure should always be kept ALARA to minimize the potential for any harm to people.
- Referring physicians should justify the need for every radiation procedure and should accept basic responsibility for protecting the patient from ionizing radiation.
- The benefits of exposing a patient to ionizing radiation should far outweigh any slight risk of inducing radiogenic cancer or genetic defects.

- Radiographers should select the smallest radiation exposure that produces the best radiographic results and should avoid errors that result in repeated radiographic exposures.
- Imaging facilities must have an effective radiation safety program that provides for patient protection and education.
- BERT is used to compare the amount of radiation a patient receives from a radiologic procedure with natural background radiation received over a specific period.
- Ionizing radiation produces electrically charged particles that can cause biologic damage on the molecular, cellular, and organic levels in human beings.
- Equivalent dose (EqD) is a quantity that attempts to take into account the variation in biologic harm produced by different types of radiation. It enables the calculation of the effective dose.
- Effective dose (EfD) takes into account the dose of all types of ionizing radiation to human organs and tissues and the weighting factor of those body parts for the development of a radiation-induced malignancy (or, for the reproductive organs, the risk of genetic damage).
- Both occupational and nonoccupational dose limits are expressed as effective dose.
- The sievert (Sv) is the International System (SI) unit and the rem is the traditional unit used to measure the EqD and the EfD.
- Sources of ionizing radiation may be natural or manmade.
  - Natural sources include radioactive materials in the earth's crust, cosmic rays from the sun and beyond the solar system, internal radiation from radionuclides deposited in human beings through natural processes, and terrestrial radiation in the environment.
  - Manmade sources include consumer products containing radioactive material, air travel, nuclear fuel, atmospheric fallout from nuclear weapons, nuclear power plant accidents, and medical radiation from diagnostic x-ray machines and radiopharmaceuticals used in nuclear medicine procedures.

Exercise 1—Crossword Puzzle

Use the clues to complete the crossword puzzle.

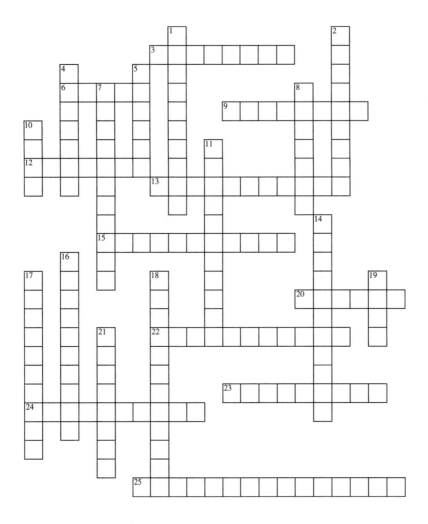

Down

1. Referring to radiation, what EqD and EfD are.
2. Location of nuclear power plant that exploded in 1986 near Kiev in the Ukraine.
4. Radiation produced by human beings (e.g., medical radiation).
5. X-ray examinations that are necessary because of technical error or carelessness.
7. Nonionizing radiation.
8. Damage to the human body resulting from significant exposure to ionizing radiation.
10. Method that compares the amount of radiation received with natural background radiations received over a given period.
11. Category of ionizing radiation that includes alpha and beta radiation.
14. Most effective tool for early diagnosis of breast cancer.
16. Dose that ultimately may be delivered from a given intake of radionuclide.
17. Effective measures used by radiation workers to safeguard patients, personnel, and the general public.
18. Radiation exposure received by a radiographer during the fulfillment of duties.
19. Possibility of inducing a radiogenic cancer or genetic defect after irradiation.
21. Radiation that produces positively and negatively charged particles when passing through matter.

Across

3. Dark spots that occasionally appear on the sun's surface.
6. Radiation exposure delivered to the whole body over a period of less than a few hours.
9. Electrically neutral components of an atom.
12. Energy that humans can safely control.
13. Type of radiation present in variable amounts in the earth's crust.
15. White blood cells that defend the body against foreign invaders.
20. Radiation of extraterrestrial origin.
22. Radiation exposure that does not benefit a person in terms of diagnostic information obtained.
23. Dose level below which individuals would have no chance of sustaining specific biologic damage.
24. Process that is the foundation of the interactions of x-rays with human tissues.
25. Electric and magnetic fields that fluctuate rapidly as they travel through space in the form of a wave.

Exercise 2—Matching

Match the following terms with their definitions or associated phrases.

1. _____ ALARA
2. _____ fallout
3. _____ electromagnetic wave
4. _____ rem
5. _____ BERT
6. _____ radiation protection
7. _____ EqD
8. _____ radionuclide
9. _____ organic damage
10. _____ diagnostic efficacy
11. _____ EfD
12. _____ genetic damage
13. _____ enhanced natural sources
14. _____ biologic effects
15. _____ protons
16. _____ Sv
17. _____ cellular damage

A. Effective measures used by radiation workers to safeguard patients, personnel, and the general public from unnecessary exposure to ionizing radiation

B. The degree to which the diagnostic study accurately reveals the presence or absence of disease in a patient

C. Traditional unit of measure for the EqD

D. Damage to living tissue of animals and human beings exposed to radiation

E. Biologic effects of ionizing radiation or other agents on generations yet unborn

F. Electric and magnetic fields that fluctuate rapidly as they travel through space, including radio waves, microwaves, visible light, and x-rays

G. Genetic or somatic changes in a living organism (e.g., mutation, cataracts, and leukemia) caused by excessive cellular damage from exposure to ionizing radiation

H. Quantity that attempts to take into account the variation in biologic harm that is produced by different types of radiation

I. Dose that takes into account the dose for all types of ionizing radiation to human organs or tissues and the overall harm (i.e., the weighting factor) of those biologic components for the development of a radiation-induced cancer (or, for the reproductive organs, the risk of genetic damage)

J. SI unit of measure for the EqD

K. Method for comparing the amount of radiation received from a radiologic procedure with natural background radiation received over a given period

L. Produces positively and negatively charged particles (ions) when passing through matter

M. The complete range of frequencies and energies of electromagnetic radiation

N. Energy in transit from one location to another

O. Injury on the cellular level caused by sufficient exposure to ionizing radiation at the molecular level

P. Acronym for as low as reasonably achievable

Q. Rays from the sun and beyond the solar system

18. _____ terrestrial radiation

R. Long-lived radioactive elements present in variable amounts in the earth's crust that emit densely ionizing radiations

19. _____ radiation

S. Consists of two protons and two neutrons

20. _____ beta particle

T. Natural sources of ionizing radiation that become increased because of accidental or deliberate human actions

21. _____ ionizing radiation

U. High speed electrons ejected from a nucleus that undergoes beta decay

22. _____ alpha particle

V. The number of protons contained within the nucleus of an atom

23. _____ electromagnetic spectrum

W. Positively charged components of an atom

24. _____ cosmic rays

X. Radiation produced as a consequence of nuclear weapons testing and chemical explosions in nuclear power plants

25. _____ atomic number

Y. An unstable nucleus that emits one or more forms of ionizing radiation to achieve greater stability

Exercise 3—Multiple Choice

Select the answer that best completes the following questions or statements.

1. Which of the following *increases* radiation exposure for both the patient and the radiographer?
   A. Production of optimal radiographs with the first exposure
   B. Use of appropriate radiation protection procedures
   C. Repeated radiographic exposures as a result of technical error or carelessness
   D. Limited radiographic examination, as ordered by the radiologist

2. To implement an effective radiation safety program in a facility that provides imaging services, the employer must provide all of the following *except:*
   A. An appropriate environment in which to execute an ALARA program and the necessary resources to support the program
   B. X-ray equipment that can produce only very low kilovoltage and very high milliamperage
   C. A written policy that describes the ALARA program and identifies management's commitment to keeping all radiation exposure as low as reasonably achievable
   D. Periodic exposure audits to determine ways to lower radiation exposure in the workplace

3. Radon accounts for approximately what percentage of the gross common exposure to human beings from natural background radiation?
   A. 15%
   B. 25%
   C. 55%
   D. 75%

4. Occupational and nonoccupational doses will remain well below maximum allowable levels when
   A. Radiographers and radiologists keep exposure as low as reasonably achievable.
   B. Referring physicians stop ordering imaging procedures.
   C. Orders for imaging procedures are determined only by medical insurance companies.
   D. Patients assume sole responsibility for ordering their imaging procedures.

5. Manmade radiation contributes what amount of mSv (mrem) to the annual exposure of the U.S. population?
   A. 0.3 (30)
   B. 0.65 (65)
   C. 1.2 (120)
   D. 3.6 (360)

6. Which of the following places human beings in closer contact with extraterrestrial radiation?
   A. Posteroanterior and lateral chest radiographs
   B. Deep-sea diving
   C. A flight on a commercial airplane
   D. Visit to a nuclear power plant

7. What do airport surveillance systems; ionization-type smoke detectors; older, luminous dial time-pieces; nuclear power plants; and false teeth made of porcelain have in common?
   A. They are all sources of natural background radiation.
   B. They each contribute 0.05 mSv (5 mrem) per year to the equivalent dose received by the global population.
   C. They are not sources of ionizing radiation.
   D. They are all sources of manmade radiation.

8. From which of the following sources do human beings receive the *largest* dose of ionizing radiation?
   A. Radioactive fallout from atomic weapons
   B. Medical radiation procedures
   C. Cosmic rays
   D. Area around a nuclear reactor

9. Medical radiation exposure from the use of diagnostic x-ray machines and radiopharmaceuticals *collectively* accounts for approximately what amount of the average annual individual effective dose of ionizing radiation?
   A. 0.25 mSv (25 mrem)
   B. 0.54 mSv (54 mrem)
   C. 0.78 mSv (78 mrem)
   D. 0.92 mSv (92 mrem)

10. Of the following groups of people, which group is most likely to suffer adverse health effects as a consequence of *substantial* exposure to ionizing radiation?
   A. Employees on duty at TMI-2 at the time of the 1979 nuclear power plant accident
   B. Members of the general population living within 50 miles of the TMI-2 nuclear reactor at the time of the 1979 accident
   C. Members of the general population living near Kiev in the former Soviet Union at the time of the 1986 accident at the Chernobyl nuclear power plant
   D. News reporters visiting the former Soviet Union 10 years after the 1986 Chernobyl accident

11. Which of the following is a radiation quantity that attempts to take into account the variation in biologic harm that is produced by different types of radiation?
   A. Absorbed dose
   B. Background equivalent radiation time
   C. Equivalent dose
   D. Exposure

12. A 3-year pilot research project was launched in the Republic of Belarus in 1996, in the aftermath of the Chernobyl nuclear accident, to empower local citizens in making their own decisions regarding reconstruction of their overall quality of life; this project was known as the
   A. ALARA Program
   B. Belarus Health Impact Study
   C. Chernobyl Rehabilitation Taskforce
   D. ETHOS Project

13. Any radiation exposure that *does not* benefit a person in terms of diagnostic information obtained or that *does not* enhance the quality of a radiologic examination is called
   A. Artificial radiation
   B. Enhanced natural background radiation
   C. Terrestrial radiation
   D. Unnecessary radiation

14. The amount of radiation a patient receives may be indicated in terms of
   1. Entrance skin exposure
   2. Bone marrow dose
   3. Gonadal dose
   A. 1 and 2 only
   B. 1 and 3 only
   C. 2 and 3 only
   D. 1, 2, and 3

15. When an imaging procedure is justified in terms of medical necessity, diagnostic efficacy is achieved when optimal radiographs revealing the presence or absence of disease are obtained with
   A. Maximal radiation exposure
   B. Minimal radiation exposure
   C. Scattered radiation exposure
   D. Secondary radiation exposure

16. Ultraviolet radiation, visible light, infrared rays, microwaves, and radio waves are considered to be nonionizing because they
   A. Have sufficient kinetic energy to eject electrons from atoms
   B. Do not have sufficient kinetic energy to eject electrons from atoms
   C. Have sufficient potential energy to eject electrons from atoms
   D. Do not have sufficient potential energy to eject electrons from atoms

17. Which of the following is a naturally occurring process by which instability of the nucleus is relieved through various types of nuclear spontaneous emissions?
   A. Electromagnetic radiation
   B. Electromagnetic ionization
   C. Radioactive decay
   D. Radioactive fallout

18. Effective radiation protection measures take into consideration
   1. Both human and environmental physical determinants
   2. Technical elements
   3. Procedural factors
   A. 1 and 2 only
   B. 1 and 3 only
   C. 2 and 3 only
   D. 1, 2, and 3

19. Radioactive elements in the earth's crust and in the human body may be classified as
   A. Enhanced natural sources of ionizing radiation
   B. Enhanced manmade sources of ionizing radiation
   C. Natural sources of ionizing radiation
   D. Unnatural sources of ionizing radiation

20. Medical radiation procedures account for
   A. The largest dose of ionizing radiation received by human beings
   B. The second largest dose of ionizing radiation received by human beings
   C. The smallest dose of ionizing radiation received by human beings
   D. Negligible doses of ionizing radiation received by human beings

21. Which of the following commonly used building materials contain(s) radon?
    A. Bricks
    B. Concrete
    C. Gypsum wallboard
    D. All of the above

22. The United States performed above-ground nuclear weapons tests before 1963. During the _____ _____, an atomic cloud was created by a 37-kiloton testing device that was exploded from a balloon at the Nevada test site on June 24, 1957. The top of the atomic cloud, which contained manmade ionizing radiation, ascended approximately 43,000 feet.
    A. Bikini Test
    B. Manhattan Project
    C. Priscilla Test
    D. Rongelap Project

23. The most effective tool(s) for diagnosing breast cancer continue to be
    A. PA and lateral chest x-rays
    B. Clinical breast self-examination
    C. Clinical breast examination by a physician
    D. Mammography

24. The millisievert (mSv), a subunit of the sievert, is equal to
    A. $^1/_{10,000}$ of a sievert
    B. $^1/_{1000}$ of a sievert
    C. $^1/_{100}$ of a sievert
    D. $^1/_{10}$ of a sievert

25. Repetition of a radiographic exposure because of poor patient positioning results in
    A. No significant change in total radiation exposure to the patient or the radiographer
    B. A slight decrease in total radiation exposure to the patient and the radiographer
    C. An increase in total radiation exposure to the patient and the radiographer
    D. A significant decrease in total radiation exposure to the patient and the radiographer

Exercise 4—True or False

Circle *T* if the statement listed below is true; circle *F* if the statement is false.

1. T F The number of protons in the nucleus of an atom constitutes the atomic number, or *A* number.

2. T F The sievert (Sv) is the SI unit of EqD.

3. T F Porcelain used for making dentures is a common example of a consumer product that contains radioactive material.

4. T F A threshold exists for radiation-induced malignant disease.

5. T F BERT is based on an annual U.S. population exposure of approximately 1 mSv per year (approximately 100 mrem per year).

6. T F Radio waves, microwaves, visible light, and x-rays are forms of electromagnetic waves.

7. T F Particulate radiations do not vary in their ability to penetrate matter.

8. T F EfD enables the calculation of the EqD.

9. T F Human beings are not continuously exposed to sources of ionizing radiation.

10. T F A significantly higher number of leukemia cases has been seen in Russian liquidators who worked at the Chernobyl power station complex in 1986 and 1987.

11. T F Atmospheric nuclear testing has escalated since 1980.

12. T F Color television monitors in use today produce substantial radiation exposure for the general public.

13. T F Most radiation-induced cancers have a latent period of 15 years or longer.

14. T F Sources of ionizing radiation may be natural or manmade.

15. T F If emitted from a radioisotope deposited in the body (e.g., in the lungs), alpha particles cannot be absorbed in epithelial tissue and therefore are not damaging to that tissue.

16. T F The average U.S. inhabitant receives an equivalent dose of approximately 0.5 mSv (50 mrem) per year from extraterrestrial radiation.

17. T F In total, the radon, cosmic ray radiations, and terrestrial and internally deposited radionuclides that comprise the natural background radiation in the United States result in an estimated average annual individual equivalent dose of approximately 2.95 mSv (295 mrem).

18. T F *Wavelength* is the distance between two consecutive crests or troughs in a wave.

19. T F An electron has approximately the same mass as a proton.

20. T F Changes in white blood cell count are a classic example of molecular damage caused by significant exposure to ionizing radiation.

21. T F Some people are exposed to a wide variety of sources of ionizing radiation, whereas others are exposed to a limited number.

22. T F Nonsmokers exposed to high radon levels have a higher risk of lung cancer than do smokers.

23. T F The solar contribution to the cosmic ray background decreases during periods of high sunspot activity.

24. T F Diagnostic efficacy is a vital part of radiation protection in the healing arts.

25. T F When radiographers use their knowledge to answer a patient's questions about the risk of radiation exposure honestly, they can do much to alleviate the patient's apprehension during a routine radiologic examination.

Exercise 5—Fill in the Blank

Fill in the blanks with the word or words that best complete the statements below.

1. The actual _____ _____ to the global population from atmospheric fallout from nuclear weapons testing is not received all at once. It is instead delivered over a period of years at changing _____ _____.

2. Most radiation-induced cancers have a ____ _____ _____ of 15 years or longer.

3. The aim of the _____ _____ is to rebuild acceptable living conditions for local citizens in contaminated territories in the Ukraine region of Russia by actively involving them in the reconstruction process.

4. When ionizing radiation is used to obtain a mammogram for the welfare of a patient, the directly realized _____ of the exposure to this radiant energy _____ _____ any slight risk of induction of a radiogenic malignancy or genetic defect.

5. In medicine, when radiation safety principles are applied correctly during imaging procedures, the _____ deposited in living tissue by radiation can be limited, thereby reducing the potential for _____ _____.

6. The quantity of _____ radiation present in any area depends on the composition of the soil or rocks in that geographic area.

7. _____ radiation consists predominantly of high-energy protons.

8. The tissues of the human body contain many naturally existing _____, which have been ingested in minute quantities from various foods or inhaled as particles in the air.

9. If a person spends 10 hours flying aboard a commercial aircraft during a period of normal sunspot activity, that individual receives a radiation _____ _____ equal to the dose received from one chest x-ray.

10. Medical radiation exposure results from the use of diagnostic _____ _____ and _____ in medicine.

11. Radiologic technologists and radiologists are educated in the _____ _____ of radiation-producing imaging equipment.

12. When ionizing radiation is used for the welfare of the patient, the directly realized _____ of exposure to radiant energy far _____ any slight _____ of induction of a radiogenic malignancy or a genetic defect.

13. The _____ concept should serve as a guide for the selection of technical radiographic and fluoroscopic exposure factors for all patient imaging procedures.

14. _____ does not imply radiation risk; it is simply a means for _____.

15. The Environmental Protection Agency (EPA) considers _____ to be the second leading cause of _____ cancer in the United States.

16. _____ in the soil and air add to the human radiation dose burden.

17. The intensity of cosmic rays varies with altitude relative to the earth's surface. The _____ intensity occurs at high altitudes, and the _____ intensity occurs at sea level.

18. Artificial teeth made in the United States are estimated to give the tissues of the oral cavity an average dose of _____ mSv/yr (_____ mrem/yr).

19. When spread over the inhabitants of the United States, fallout from nuclear weapons tests and other environmental sources contributes less than _____ mSv (_____ mrem) annually to the equivalent dose of each person.

20. _____ cancer continues to be the main adverse health effect of the 1986 accident at the Chernobyl nuclear power plant.

21. Referring physicians should _____ the need for every radiation procedure and accept the

7

basic _____ for protecting the patient from ionizing radiation.

22. Ionizing radiation has both a _____ and a _____ potential.

23. During the accident at the TMI-2 nuclear power plant in March, 1979, the U.S. Department of Energy estimated that about _____% of the material in the TMI-2 nuclear reactor core reached a _____ state.

24. In cooler months, when homes and buildings are tightly closed, radon levels are usually _____.

25. The full range of _____ and _____ of electromagnetic waves is known as the *electromagnetic spectrum*.

Exercise 6—Labeling

Label the following illustrations and table.

A. X-ray tube.

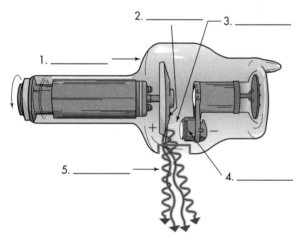

B. Percentage contribution of each natural and manmade radiation source to the total average effective dose for inhabitants of the United States.

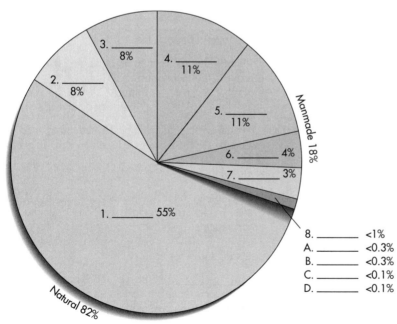

From National Council on Radiation Protection and Measurements (NCRP): *Report No. 93, ionizing radiation exposure of the population of the United States,* Bethesda, MD, 1987, The Council.

C. Radiation equivalent dose and subsequent biologic effects of acute whole body exposure*

Radiation Equivalent Dose (EqD)	Subsequent Biologic Effect
1. ___ Sv (___ rem)	Blood changes (e.g., measurable hematologic depression, decreases in the number of lymphocytes present in the circulating blood)
2. ___ Sv (___ rem)	Nausea, diarrhea
3. ___ Sv (___ rem)	Erythema (diffuse redness over an area of skin after irradiation)
4. ___ Sv (___ rem)	If dose is to gonads, temporary sterility
5. ___ Sv (___ rem)	50% chance of death; lethal dose for 50% of population over 30 days (LD 50/30)
6. ___ Sv (___ rem)	Death

*Radiation exposures are delivered to the entire body over a time period of less than a few hours.
Modified from Radiologic health, unit 4, slide 17, Denver, Multi-Media Publishing (slide program).

Exercise 7—Short Answer
Answer the following questions by providing a short answer.

1. How can human beings exercise greater control over the use of radiant energy?

_____

_____

2. How can radiologic technologists reduce radiation exposure to patients and to themselves?

_____

_____

3. How does ionizing radiation damage normal biologic tissue?

_____

_____

4. What is the basis of the concept of radiation dose?

_____

_____

5. Describe what can happen to a living organism if excessive cellular damage occurs as a consequence of radiation exposure.

_____

_____

6. What is the origin of cosmic radiation? From what does it result?

_____

_____

7. Name four radionuclides found in small quantities in the human body.

_____

_____

Chapter 1 **Introduction to Radiation Protection**

8. Why is it impossible to estimate accurately the total annual equivalent dose from fallout?

_____

_____

9. How is risk weighed against benefit in medical radiography?

_____

_____

10. Why does the patient dose for each x-ray examination vary from one health care facility to another?

_____

_____

11. List six consequences of ionization in human cells.

_____

_____

12. What actually produces the sensation of heat or the chemical changes that produce suntan and sunburn?

_____

_____

13. What subunit of the rem is equal to $^{1}/_{1000}$ of a rem?

_____

_____

14. List six sources of manmade, or artificial, ionizing radiation.

_____

_____

15. List three advantages of using the BERT method to compare the amount of radiation received with the natural background radiation received over a given period.

_____

_____

16. What disease continues to be the main adverse health effect of the 1986 accident at the Chernobyl nuclear power plant?

_____

_____

17. List three ways to indicate the amount of radiation received by a patient.

_____

_____

18. What radiation quantity enables the calculation of the effective dose?

_____

_____

19. What is kinetic energy?

_____

_____

20. In terms of ability to penetrate biologic matter, how do alpha particles compare with beta particles? Why are alpha particles considered virtually harmless as an external source of radiation?

_____

_____

Exercise 8—Essay
On a separate sheet of paper, answer the following questions in essay form.

1. What have been the mental and physical effects of the 1979 accident at the TMI-2 nuclear power plant on occupationally exposed individuals and on the people living in communities near the plant?

2. What mental and adverse physical health effects have been attributed to the 1986 disaster at the Chernobyl nuclear power plant from the time of the accident to now? Discuss the consequences of this accident for plant workers, the exposed population, and the remaining global population.

3. Discuss the significance of the ETHOS Project and explain the value of this program to the community in the Republic of Belarus.

4. How can a radiographer maintain radiation exposure ALARA on a daily basis in a clinical setting?

5. Using the information in Table 1-2 in the text, compare the use, frequency, wavelength, and energy of the radiations that make up the electromagnetic spectrum.

6. Describe the value of patient education with regard to radiation procedures and radiation safety.

7. Discuss the importance of diagnostic efficacy as it relates to medical x-ray procedures and radiation safety for the patient.

8. Discuss the responsibility of the employer in a health care facility for maintaining the ALARA concept in the workplace.

9. Applying the concept of BERT, explain how a radiographer might respond to a patient who asks how much radiation he or she will receive from a routine x-ray series of the lumbar spine.

10. Describe the health impact of radon exposure in human beings.

The student should take this test after reading Chapter 1, finishing all accompanying textbook and workbook exercises, and completing any additional activities required by the course instructor. The student should complete the post test with a score of 90% or higher before advancing to the next chapter. (Each of the following 20 questions or blanks is worth 5 points.) Score = _____ %

1. Define the term *radiation protection.*

_____

_____

2. What term (and acronym) is used to express the concept of keeping radiation exposure to a level that minimizes the potential for damage to human tissue?

_____

3. Who should justify the need for every radiation procedure and accept basic responsibility for protecting the patient from ionizing radiation?

_____

4. The benefits of exposing patients to ionizing radiation should far outweigh any slight _____ of induction of radiogenic cancer or genetic defects.

5. What must imaging facilities have that provides for patient protection and patient education?

_____

6. What does ionizing radiation produce that can cause biologic damage on the molecular, cellular, and organic levels in human beings?

_____

7. Both occupational and nonoccupational dose limits are expressed as _____ dose.

8. What are the SI unit and the traditional unit of measure for the EqD and the EfD?

_____

_____

9. Which of the following radiation quantities takes into account the dose of all types of ionizing radiation to human organs and tissues and the weighting factor of those body parts for the development of a radiation-induced malignancy (or, for the reproductive organs, the risk of genetic damage)?
   A. Absorbed dose
   B. Effective dose
   C. Equivalent dose
   D. Exposure

10. Any radiation exposure that does not benefit a person in terms of diagnostic information obtained or that does not enhance the quality of a radiologic examination is called:
   A. Enhanced natural background radiation
   B. Environmental radiation
   C. Manmade radiation
   D. Unnecessary radiation

11. Entrance skin exposure (ESE), bone marrow dose, and gonadal dose may be used to indicate

_____

12. What is the term used for the full range of frequencies and wavelengths of electromagnetic waves?

_____

13. The radioactive elements in the earth's crust and in the human body are considered what type of sources of ionizing radiation?

_____

14. What method can a radiographer use to compare the amount of radiation received for a routine radiographic procedure with natural background radiation received over a given period?

_____

15. The EPA considers the second leading cause of lung cancer in the United States to be:
A. Diagnostic x-rays
B. Normal exposure to natural background radiation
C. Radon
D. Cosmic rays

16. Which of the following is a consumer product that contains radioactive material?
   1. Porcelain used to make dentures
   2. Airport surveillance systems
   3. Video display terminals that use cathode ray tubes
A. 1 and 2 only
B. 1 and 3 only
C. 2 and 3 only
D. 1, 2, and 3

17. Are alpha particles more harmful as an external source of radiation or as an internal source of radiation?

_____

18. Radiographers should select the smallest radiation exposure that produces the best radiographic results and should avoid errors that result in _____ radiographic exposures.

19. What disease continues to be the main adverse health effect of the 1986 accident at the Chernobyl nuclear power plant?

_____

20. Radiation damage to generations yet unborn defines _____.

2 Interaction of X-Radiation with Matter

Chapter 2 covers the basic concepts of physics that relate to radiation absorption and scatter. The processes of interaction between radiation and matter are emphasized to provide the background that allows radiographers to select the optimal technical exposure factors, such as the peak kilovoltage (kVp) and the milliampere-seconds (mAs). Selection of the appropriate techniques can minimize the radiation dose to the patient and produce radiographs of acceptable quality.

CHAPTER HIGHLIGHTS

- Biologic damage in the patient may result from absorption of x-ray energy.
- Variations in the x-ray absorption properties of various body structures makes radiographic imaging of human anatomy possible.
- *Attenuation* results when, through the process of absorption and scatter, the intensity of the primary photons of an x-ray beam decreases as it passes through matter.
- Scattered radiation can result in radiographic fog or can be a biologic hazard to the radiographer.
- The energy absorbed by the patient per unit mass is called the *absorbed dose.*
- Two interactions of x-radiation are important in diagnostic radiology: photoelectric absorption and Compton scattering. The photoelectric effect is the basis of radiographic imaging, whereas the Compton effect is its bane.
- For each radiographic procedure, an optimal kVp and mAs combination exists that minimizes the dose to the patient and produces an acceptable radiograph.
  - Within the energy range of diagnostic radiology that includes mammography (23 to 150 kVp), when kVp is decreased, the number of photoelectric interactions increases and the number of Compton interactions decreases; however, more energy is absorbed by the patient, and the patient dose is increased.
  - When kVp is increased, the patient receives a lower dose, but image quality is compromised.
  - kVp selection usually is based on the type of procedure and body part to be radiographed.
- Radiographers must balance other variables, such as film-screen combination, patient thickness, and the degree of muscle tissue, to arrive at technical exposure factors that provide an acceptable image within the standards of radiation protection.
- Coherent scattering is most likely to occur below a 30 kVp generator setting; pair production and photodisintegration occur far above the range of diagnostic radiology.

15

Exercise 1—Crossword Puzzle

Use the clues to complete the crossword puzzle.

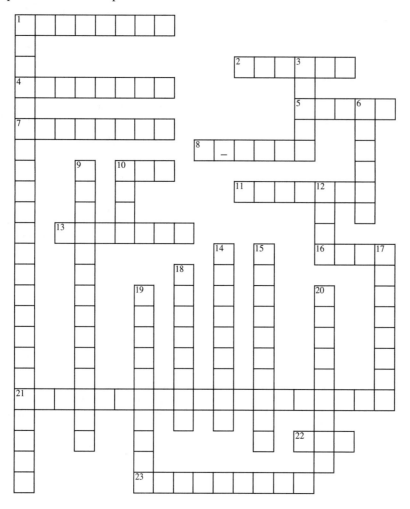

Down

1. Most important mode of interaction between photons and the atoms of the patient's body for producing useful patient images.
3. Type of window in the x-ray tube that permits passage of all but the lowest energy components of the x-ray beam.
6. Type of transmission that occurs when some x-ray photons traverse an object without interacting.
9. Radiation released as a result of a photoelectric interaction between an x-ray photon and an atom.
10. Type of radiographic image receptor.
12. Seconds, during which the x-ray tube is activated.
14. Unit of measure meaning thousands of volts.
15. Type of scattered radiation that degrades the appearance of a finished radiograph by blurring the sharp patterns of dense objects.
17. Metal with a high melting point and high atomic number that the target of an x-ray tube is made of.
18. Type of damage in the patient that may result from the absorption of x-rays.
19. Another name for coherent scattering.
20. Type of atomic number that is a composite Z number for many different chemical elements composing a material.

Across

1. Form of antimatter.
2. A most common method devised to limit the effects of indirectly transmitted x-ray photons.
4. Scattering that occurs when a low-energy photon interacts with one or more free electrons.
5. Target of an x-ray tube.
7. Person responsible for the theory mathematically expressed as $E = mc^2$.
8. Radiation that has neither mass nor electric charge and that travels at the speed of light.
10. Undesirable additional density on an x-ray film that can be caused by scattered radiation.
11. Type of energy an x-ray photon possesses.
13. Radiation that emerges directly from the x-ray tube collimator and moves without deflection toward a wall, door, viewing window, and so on.
16. All of the x-ray photons that reach the image receptor.
21. Process of interaction of x-ray with matter that does not occur within the range of diagnostic radiology.
22. Controls the quality, or penetrating power, of the photons in the x-ray beam.
23. What happens to patient dose when kVp is increased.

Exercise 2—Matching

Match the following terms with their definitions or associated phrases.

1. _____ absorption
2. _____ permanent inherent filtration
3. _____ photoelectric absorption
4. _____ fluorescent yield
5. _____ mAs
6. _____ kVp
7. _____ deuteron
8. _____ Compton scattering
9. _____ effective atomic number (Zeff)
10. _____ aluminum
11. _____ positron
12. _____ radiographic fog
13. _____ attenuation
14. _____ radiographic density
15. _____ photoelectron
16. _____ rhenium tungsten
17. _____ pair production
18. _____ 13.8
19. _____ annihilation radiation

A. Reduction in the number of photons in the x-ray beam through absorption
B. Effective atomic number of compact bone
C. Interaction of an x-ray photon with a loosely bound outer shell electron of an atom
D. Product of electron tube current and the time (in seconds) the x-ray tube is on
E. Effective atomic number of soft tissue
F. The anode of an x-ray tube can be made of this metal
G. Transference of electromagnetic energy to the atoms of a material
H. Byproduct of photoelectric interaction
I. Undesirable, additional density on an x-ray film
J. Proton-neutron combination
K. Interaction between an x-ray photon and an inner shell electron of an atom
L. Metal that hardens the x-ray beam by removing low-energy components
M. The highest energy level of photons in the x-ray beam
N. Positively charged electron
O. Combination of the x-ray tube glass wall and the added aluminum placed in the collimator
P. Refers to the number of characteristic x-rays emitted per inner shell vacancy
Q. A composite Z for a material that consists of different chemical elements
R. The degree of overall blackening on the finished radiograph
S. Interaction in which the energy of the incoming photon is transformed into two new particles, a negatron and a positron

20. _____ E = mc²

T. Radiation in the form of two oppositely moving 511 keV photons generated as the result of mutual annihilation of matter and antimatter

21. _____ 7.4

U. Mathematical expression of Einstein's theory of relativity

22. _____ absorbed dose

V. Energy absorbed by the patient per unit mass

23. _____ x-ray photons

W. All of the x-ray photons that reach their destination (the image receptor) after passing through the object being radiographed

24. _____ negative contrast media

X. These agents result in darker areas on the processed radiograph

25. _____ image formation radiation

Y. Particles associated with electromagnetic radiation that have neither mass nor charge and that travel at the speed of light

Exercise 3—Multiple Choice

Select the answer that best completes the following questions or statements.

1. When a technical exposure factor of 90 kVp is selected, which of the following occurs?
   A. The energy of the highest energy photon in the x-ray beam is 30 keV.
   B. The electrons are accelerated from the cathode to the anode with an energy of 30 keV.
   C. The energy of the average photon in the x-ray beam is 90 keV.
   D. The energy of the average photon in the x-ray beam is 30 keV.

2. The passage of x-ray photons through an object *without* interaction is called
   A. Absorption
   B. Attenuation
   C. Scattering
   D. Direct transmission

3. In which of the following x-ray interactions with matter is the energy of the incident photon *completely* absorbed?
   A. Compton
   B. Photoelectric
   C. Incoherent
   D. Rayleigh

4. What is the result of coherent scattering?
   A. Usually just a small angle change in the direction of the incident photon
   B. Transfer of all energy of the incident x-ray photon to the atoms of the irradiated object
   C. Production of a negatron and a positron
   D. Transfer of only some of the energy of the incident x-ray photon to the atoms of the irradiated object

5. A technical exposure factor of 100 kVp means that the electrons bombarding the anode of the x-ray tube have a *maximum* energy of
   A. 1000 electron volt (eV), or 1 keV
   B. 10,000 eV, or 10 keV
   C. 100,000 eV, or 100 keV
   D. 1,000,000 eV, or 1000 keV

6. A Compton-scattered electron
   A. Annihilates another electron
   B. Is absorbed within a few microns of the site of the original Compton interaction
   C. Causes pair production
   D. Engages in the process of photodisintegration

7. Most scattered radiation produced during radiographic procedures is the *direct* result of which of the following?
   A. Photoelectric absorption
   B. Nuclear decay
   C. Image-formation electrons
   D. Compton interactions

8. A reduction in the number of primary photons in the x-ray beam through absorption and scatter as the beam passes through the object in its path defines
   A. Annihilation
   B. Attenuation
   C. Photodisintegration
   D. Radiographic fog

9. *Before* it interacts with matter, an incoming x-ray photon may be referred to as which of the following?
   A. Attenuated photon
   B. Primary photon
   C. Ionized photon
   D. Scattered photon

10. Within the energy range of diagnostic radiology that includes mammography (23 to 150 kVp), when kVp is *decreased,* the patient dose
    A. Decreases
    B. Increases
    C. Remains the same
    D. Doubles

11. Which of the following statements *best* describes mass density?
    A. It is the number of electrons per gram of tissue.
    B. It is the same as radiographic density.
    C. It relates the way the effective atomic number of biologic tissues influences absorption.
    D. It is measured in grams per cubic centimeter.

12. Of the following interactions between x-radiation and matter, which *does not* occur in the range of diagnostic radiology?
    1. Photoelectric absorption
    2. Pair production
    3. Photodisintegration
    A. 1 and 2 only
    B. 1 and 3 only
    C. 2 and 3 only
    D. 1, 2, and 3

13. For a diagnostic radiologic examination, the selection of technical exposure factors using an *optimal* kVp and mAs combination
    A. Produces an x-ray of acceptable quality but increases the patient dose
    B. Produces an x-ray of acceptable quality while minimizing the patient dose
    C. Produces an x-ray of acceptable quality without affecting the patient dose
    D. Affects neither the quality of the finished radiograph nor the patient dose

14. The quality, or penetrating power, of an x-ray beam is controlled by
    A. The absorption characteristics of the object radiographed
    B. Fluorescent yield
    C. mAs
    D. kVp

15. Small angle scatter
    A. Degrades the appearance of a finished radiograph by blurring the sharp outlines of dense objects
    B. Enhances the appearance of a finished radiograph by clearly delineating the sharp outlines of dense objects
    C. Affects the appearance of a finished radiograph only when contrast medium is used for visualization of a tissue or structure
    D. Occurs only in therapeutic radiologic ranges

16. Within the energy range of diagnostic radiology, as absorption in biologic tissue increases, the potential for biologic damage
    A. Decreases slightly
    B. Decreases significantly
    C. Increases
    D. Remains the same

17. Which of the following terms are synonymous?
    1. Coherent scattering
    2. Classical scattering
    3. Unmodified scattering
    A. 1 and 2 only
    B. 1 and 3 only
    C. 2 and 3 only
    D. 1, 2, and 3

18. Noninteracting and small angle scattered photons comprise
    A. Absorbed photons
    B. Attenuated photons
    C. Exit, or image formation, radiation
    D. Compton scatter

19. *Direct transmission* means that x-ray photons
    A. Are absorbed in biologic tissue upon interaction
    B. Are scattered upon interaction with biologic tissue
    C. Pass through biologic tissue without interaction
    D. Pass through biologic tissue with some interaction

20. Which of the following has the same mass and magnitude of charge as a negatron?
    A. Deuteron
    B. Neutron
    C. Positron
    D. Proton

21. Which of the following interactions between x-radiation and matter *does not* occur within the range of diagnostic radiology?
    A. Coherent scattering
    B. Compton scattering
    C. Photoelectric absorption
    D. Pair production

22. kVp controls
    A. Absorption characteristics of the object radiographed
    B. Fluorescent yield
    C. Random interaction of x-ray photons with the image receptor
    D. Quality, or penetrating power, of the photons in the x-ray beam

23. *Primary radiation* is synonymous with
    A. Direct radiation
    B. Compton scatter
    C. Elastic scatter
    D. Rayleigh radiation

24. Which of the following are radiographic image receptors?
    1. Radiographic grid
    2. Phosphorescent screen
    3. X-ray film
    A. 1 and 2 only
    B. 1 and 3 only
    C. 2 and 3 only
    D. 1, 2, and 3

25. The process most responsible for the contrast between bone and soft tissue in diagnostic radiographs is
    A. Coherent scattering
    B. Compton scattering
    C. Photoelectric absorption
    D. Photodisintegration

Exercise 4—True or False

Circle *T* if the statement listed below is true; circle *F* if the statement is false.

1. T F The radiographer also benefits when the patient dose is minimal because less radiation is scattered from the patient.

2. T F The optimum x-ray image is formed when only indirect transmission photons reach the image receptor.

3. T F Coherent scattering does not contribute to radiographic fog in mammography because breast tissue is gently but firmly compressed during this imaging procedure.

4. T F During the process of Compton scattering, an x-ray photon interacts with an inner shell electron of an atom of the irradiated object.

5. T F A photoelectron usually is absorbed within a few micrometers of the biologic tissue, thereby increasing the patient dose.

6. T F Absorption properties between different body structures must be identical to make diagnostically useful radiographs possible.

7. T F The intensity of radiation scatter in various directions is a major factor in the planning of protection for medical imaging personnel during a radiologic examination.

8. T F Pair production is also known as Rayleigh scattering.

9. T F In the radiographic kilovoltage range, compact bone with a high calcium content by weight undergoes much more photoelectric absorption than an equal mass of soft tissue and air.

10. T F The use of positive contrast media leads to a decrease in absorbed dose in the body structures that contain it.

11. T F Compton scattering results in all-directional scatter.

12. T F A Compton-scattered electron is also known as an *Auger electron.*

13. T F Rayleigh and Thompson types of scattering play essentially no role in radiography.

14. T F For each radiographic procedure, an optimal kVp and mAs combination exists that minimizes the dose to the patient and produces an acceptable radiograph.

15. T F A photoelectron may interact with other atoms, but it cannot cause excitation or ionization of those atoms.

16. T F *Attenuation* is any process that increases the intensity of the primary photon beam directed toward a destination.

17. T F During the process of photoelectric absorption, the atom also emits primary radiation when the outer shell electron fills the inner shell vacancy.

18. T F The minimum energy required to produce an electron-positron pair is 0.022 megaelectron volts (MeV).

19. T F The target in the x-ray tube is also known as the *cathode.*

20. T F If an electron is drawn across an electrical potential difference of 1 volt (V), it has acquired an energy of 1 eV.

21. T F The term *exit photons* is synonymous with the term *image formation photons.*

22. T F The byproducts of photoelectric absorption include photoelectrons and characteristic x-ray photons.

23. T F The effective atomic number of air is 13.8.

24. T F Biologic damage in the patient may result from the absorption of x-ray energy.

25. T F kVp selection usually is based on the type of procedure and body part to be radiographed.

Chapter **2** **Interaction of X-Radiation with Matter**

Exercise 5—Fill in the Blank

Fill in the blanks with the word or words that best complete the statements below.

1. X-rays are carriers of _____, electromagnetic energy.

2. As _____ interact with the atoms of the target, x-ray _____ emerge from the target with a broad range of energies and leave the x-ray tube through a glass window.

3. The energy of the electrons inside the x-ray tube is expressed in terms of the _____ _____ applied across the tube.

4. In clinical situations, scattered photons reach the image receptor and _____ image quality.

5. In a diagnostic x-ray beam, the ultimate destination of photons is the _____ receptor.

6. In the process of _____ scattering, because the wavelengths of both incident and scattered waves are the same, no net energy has been absorbed by the atom.

7. Compton scatter may be directed _____ _____ as small angle scatter, _____ as backscatter, and to the side as sidescatter.

8. _____ scattering and _____ absorption in tissue are equally probable at about 35 keV.

9. An alternative to the emission of a characteristic photon is a process in which the energy that would have appeared as a photon is used instead to eject an outer shell electron. Unbound electrons generated in this manner are known as _____ electrons.

10. Biologic damage may result from the ____ _____ of x-ray energy.

11. A diagnostic x-ray beam is produced when a stream of high-speed _____ bombard a _____-charged target in a highly evacuated glass tube.

12. Although all photons in a diagnostic x-ray beam do not have the same _____, the most energetic photons in the beam can have no more

_____ than the electrons that bombard the target.

13. For a typical diagnostic x-ray unit, the energy of the average photon in the x-ray beam is about _____ _____ the energy of the most energetic photon.

14. The _____ of radiation scatter in various directions is a major factor in the planning of protection for medical imaging personnel during a radiologic examination.

15. _____ and _____ scattering play essentially no role in radiography.

16. The less a given structure attenuates radiation, the _____ will be its image on the finished radiograph.

17. Use of a positive contrast medium leads to an _____ in absorbed dose in the body structures that contain the medium.

18. A positron is classified as a form of ____ _____.

19. The _____ effect is the basis of radiographic imaging, whereas the ____ _____ effect is its bane.

20. _____ scattering is most likely to occur below a 30 kVp generator setting.

21. When _____ is increased, the patient receives a lower radiation dose, but image quality is compromised.

22. Within the energy range of diagnostic radiology that includes mammography (23 to 150 kVp), when kVp is decreased, the number of photoelectric interactions _____ and the number of Compton interactions _____; however, more energy is absorbed by the patient, and the patient dose is _____.

23. Variations in the x-ray _____ properties of various body structures make radiographic imaging of human anatomy possible.

24. A Compton-scattered electron is also known as a _____ electron.

25. An incoming x-ray photon has _____ energy.

Chapter **2** Interaction of X-Radiation with Matter

Label the following illustrations.

A. Primary, exit, and attenuated photons.

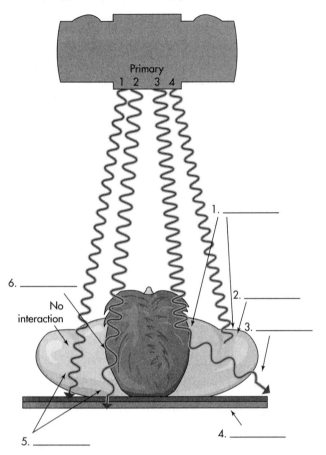

Primary
1 2 3 4

6. _____

No
interaction

1. _____

2. _____

3. _____

4. _____

5. _____

Primary − Exit = Attenuation

B. Process of Compton scattering.

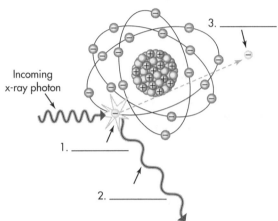

Incoming
x-ray photon

3. _____

1. _____

2. _____

C. Process of photoelectric absorption.

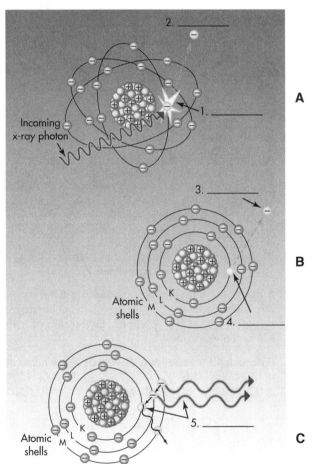

2. _____

Incoming
x-ray photon

1. _____

A

3. _____

Atomic
shells

K
L
M

4. _____

B

Atomic
shells

K
L
M

5. _____

C

Exercise 7—Short Answer

Answer the following questions by providing a short answer.

1. Name five types of interaction that can occur between x-radiation and matter.

_____

_____

2. How is a radiographer actually responsible for a dose the patient receives during an x-ray procedure?

_____

_____

3. What phenomenon is responsible for producing diagnostically useful radiographs in which different anatomic structures can be perceived and distinguished?

_____

_____

4. How can the radiographer reduce the amount of radiographic fog produced by small angle scatter?

_____

_____

5. How is the energy of the electrons inside a diagnostic x-ray tube expressed?

_____

_____

6. What is the minimum energy required to produce an electron-positron pair?

_____

_____

7. What is a positive contrast medium?

_____

_____

8. Name three unstable nuclei used in positron emission tomography (PET) scanning.

_____

_____

9. What type of energy does a photoelectron have?

_____

_____

Chapter **2** **Interaction of X-Radiation with Matter**

10. What can result from the production of scattered radiation?

_____

_____

11. List the two methods most commonly used to limit the effects of indirectly transmitted x-ray photons.

_____

_____

12. During the process of coherent scattering, why is no net energy absorbed by the atom with which the incident x-ray photon interacted?

_____

_____

13. What is mass density? How is it measured?

_____

_____

14. What is radiographic contrast?

_____

_____

15. In what radiation modality is annihilation radiation used?

_____

_____

Exercise 8—Essay

On a separate sheet of paper, answer the following questions in essay form.

1. Discuss the importance of photoelectric absorption in radiography. Explain the impact of this x-ray interaction on the patient dose.

2. Explain how a radiographer can limit the production of scattered radiation in a radiography room.

3. Discuss the use of positive contrast media in radiography. How does the use of such media affect the patient dose?

4. Discuss the probability of photon interaction with matter.

5. Explain how radiographers can select technical exposure factors for routine x-ray procedures that minimize the radiation dose to the patient and produce a radiograph of acceptable quality.

POST TEST

The student should take this test after reading Chapter 2, finishing all accompanying textbook and workbook exercises, and completing any additional activities required by the course instructor. The student should complete the post test with a score of 90% or higher before advancing to the next chapter. (Each of the following 20 questions or blanks is worth 5 points.) Score = _____ %

1. Use of a barium- or iodine-based contrast medium significantly enhances the occurrence of _____ _____ absorption in biologic tissue, resulting in an increase in the radiation dose to the patient.

2. Define the term *attenuation*.

   _____

   _____

3. For each radiographic procedure, an optimal kVp and mAs combination exists that _____ the dose to the patient and produces an acceptable radiograph.

4. Compton-scattered photons contribute significantly to the exposure of the _____.

5. During the process of Compton scattering, the energy of the incident x-ray photon is _____ absorbed.

6. What controls the quality, or penetrating power, of an x-ray beam?

   _____

7. The interaction of x-ray photons with any atoms of biologic matter are _____ in nature, therefore the effects of such interactions cannot be predicted with certainty.

8. Pair production and _____ do not occur within the range of diagnostic radiology.

9. Which interaction of x-radiation with matter is most responsible for the contrast between bone and soft tissue that is seen on an optimal quality radiograph?

   _____

10. Scattered radiation can result in
    1. A biologic hazard to the patient
    2. A biologic hazard to the radiographer
    3. Radiographic fog
    A. 1 and 2 only
    B. 1 and 3 only
    C. 2 and 3 only
    D. 1, 2, and 3

11. A positron is considered
    A. A form of antimatter
    B. A modified proton
    C. A form of small angle scatter
    D. A byproduct of the photoelectric interaction

12. The symbol *Zeff* indicates
    A. Atomic number
    B. Effective atomic number
    C. Mass number
    D. The number of vacancies in an atomic shell

13. Below a 30 kVp generator setting, which of the following x-radiation interactions with matter is most likely to occur?
    A. Coherent scattering
    B. Compton scattering
    C. Photoelectric absorption
    D. Pair production

14. Which of the following terms are synonymous?
    A. Classical scattering and photoelectric absorption
    B. Compton scattering and photodisintegration
    C. Photoelectric absorption and Compton scattering
    D. Characteristic radiation and fluorescent radiation

15. PET makes use of
    A. Annihilation radiation
    B. Compton-scattered photons
    C. Photoelectrons
    D. Bremsstrahlung

16. What is the effective atomic number of compact bone?

_____

17. What term is used for the energy absorbed by the patient per unit mass?

_____

18. To ensure the quality of the radiographic image and the patient's safety, both the radiologist and the radiographer should choose the highest energy x-ray beam that permits adequate radiographic _____.

19. Compton scattering results in _____ scatter.

20. To what does the term *fluorescent yield* refer?

_____

3 | Radiation Quantities and Units

Chapter 3 covers the evolution of radiation quantities and units. It also points up the efforts of medical professionals, ever since the harmful effects of x-rays became clear, to find a way to reduce radiation exposure throughout the world by developing standards for measuring and limiting such exposure. Diagnostic imaging personnel must be familiar with these standardized radiation quantities and units so that they can measure patient and personnel exposure consistently and uniformly.

CHAPTER HIGHLIGHTS

- Radiation units can be expressed in the International System of Units (SI) or the traditional system.
- Coulomb per kilogram (C/kg) or roentgen (R) is used for exposure in air only.
- Gray (Gy) or rad is used for the absorbed dose (D) measurement.
- Equivalent dose (EqD) and effective dose (EfD) are the quantities of choice for measuring biologic effects when all types of radiation must be considered.

- EqD specifies how much biologic damage from different types and doses of radiation will be equivalent if correct weighting factors are included.
- EfD describes the way the same effective amount of damage can be attained by giving different equivalent doses to different organs.
- Sievert (Sv) and rem are the units used to calculate the radiation quantities, EqD and EfD.
- Collective effective dose (ColEfD) is used in the calculation of group or population radiation exposure arising from low doses of different sources of ionizing radiation.
- The person-sievert is the unit used to calculate the radiation quantity, ColEfD.
- The equation for calculating the EqD is $EqD = D \times W_R$ (W_R is the radiation weighting factor).
- The equation for calculating the EfD is $EfD = D \times W_R \times W_T$ (W_T is the tissue weighting factor).

27

Exercise 1—Crossword Puzzle

Use the clues to complete the crossword puzzle.

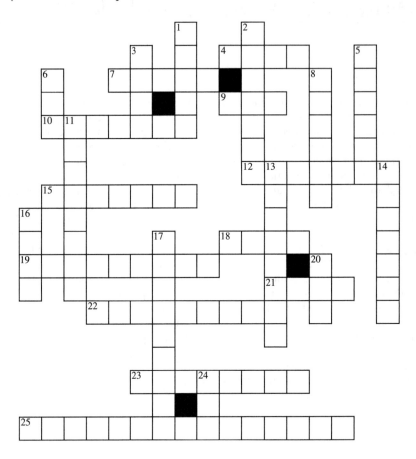

Down

1. First American radiation fatality.
2. Biologic effects of ionizing radiation, or other agents, on generations yet unborn.
3. Greek word meaning body.
5. Weighting factor that is a conceptual measure for the relative risk associated with irradiation of different body tissues.
6. Unit of energy and work.
8. Fluoroscope inventor.
11. Total electrical charge per unit mass that x-ray and gamma ray photons with energies up to 3MeV generate in dry air at standard temperatures and pressure.
13. Traditional unit of the radiation quantity, exposure (X).
14. Swedish physicist for who the SI unit of equivalent dose was named.
16. Type of somatic effect of ionizing radiation that appears months or years following exposure.
17. Radiation exposure to which occupationally exposed persons could be continuously subjected without any apparent harmful acute effects such as erythema of the skin.
20. Acronym for radiation absorbed dose.
24. Acronym for radiation-equivalent-man.

Across

4. Safe dose of ionizing radiation.
7. The work done or energy expended when a force of 1 newton acts on an object along a distance of 1 meter.
9. Concept that helps explain the need for a quality, or modifying, factor.
10. Country in which x-rays were discovered.
12. Pear-shaped, partial vacuum discharge tube.
15. Basic unit of electrical charge.
18. Part of human body imaged on the world's first x-ray picture on film.
19. Dose of radiation below which an individual has a negligible chance of sustaining specific biologic damage.
21. SI unit of D.
22. Dose that provides a measure of the overall risk of exposure to ionizing radiation.
23. Patient's skin surface where radiation dose received will be highest.
25. Condition of the skin developed by early radiologists and dentists caused by exposure to ionizing radiation.

Exercise 2—Matching

Match the following terms with their definitions or associated phrases.

1. _____ aplastic anemia

2. _____ linear energy transfer (LET)

3. _____ SI

4. _____ leukemia

5. _____ rad

6. _____ somatic damage

7. _____ Gy

8. _____ rem

9. _____ R

10. _____ person-sievert

11. _____ W_R

12. _____ occupational exposure

13. _____ EfD

14. _____ Crookes tube

15. _____ gamma radiation

16. _____ skin erythema dose

17. _____ EqD

18. _____ *soma*

19. _____ Sv

20. _____ D

21. _____ Bragg-Gray theory

22. _____ barium platinocyanide

23. _____ exposure

24. _____ traditional units

25. _____ effective atomic number (Zeff)

A. Unit used from 1900 to 1930 to measure radiation exposure

B. Traditional unit used for radiation protection purposes

C. Allows units to be used interchangeably among all branches of science throughout the world

D. Concept that helps explain the need for a quality, or modifying, factor

E. Traditional unit used to express D

F. SI unit of EqD

G. Blood disorder that results in abnormal overproduction of white blood cells following exposure to ionizing radiation

H. The product of $D \times W_R \times W_T$

I. Relates the ionization produced in a small cavity within an irradiated medium or object to the energy absorbed in that medium as a result of its radiation exposure

J. Blood disorder that results from bone marrow failure following exposure to ionizing radiation

K. Product of $D \times W_R$

L. Biologic damage to the body caused by exposure to ionizing radiation

M. SI unit for the radiation quantity, ColEfD

N. Radiation exposure received by workers while performing their professional responsibilities

O. SI unit used to express D

P. Body

Q. The amount of ionizing radiation that may strike an object (e.g., the human body) when in the vicinity of a radiation source

R. Special units associated with radiation protection and dosimetry, namely the roentgen and the rem.

S. A dimensionless factor (a multiplier) used for radiation protection to account for differences in biologic impact between various types of ionizing radiation

T. A pear-shaped, partial vacuum discharge tube

U. Fluorescent material that coated the paper used when x-rays were discovered

V. A composite, or weighted average, of the atomic numbers of the many different chemical elements that make up biologic tissue

W. Short wavelength, higher energy electromagnetic waves emitted by the nuclei of radioactive substances

X. The amount of energy per unit mass absorbed by an irradiated object

Y. The photon (either x-ray or gamma ray) exposure that, under standard conditions of pressure and temperature, produces a total positive or negative ion charge of 2.58×10^{-4} C/kg of dry air

29

Exercise 3—Multiple Choice

Select the answer that best completes the following questions or statements.

1. Which of the following factors must be multiplied to determine the EfD from an x-radiation exposure to an organ or body part?
   A. $EqD \times W_R \times D$
   B. $W_T \times W_R \times ColEfD$
   C. $D \times W_R \times W_T$
   D. $D \times C/kg$

2. Which of the following is the SI unit of radiation exposure?
   A. C/kg
   B. Gy
   C. R
   D. Sv

3. The expression 10^{-6} may be *symbolically* expressed as which of the following?
   A. π
   B. Ω
   C. Σ
   D. μ

4. In radiation protection systems no longer in use, a radiation dose to which occupationally exposed persons could be continuously subjected *without* any apparent harmful acute effects (e.g., erythema of the skin) was known as a(n)
   A. Effective dose
   B. Maximum permissible dose
   C. Tolerance dose
   D. Weighted dose

5. Short-term somatic effects of radiation include
   1. Nausea and fatigue
   2. Blood and intestinal disorders
   3. Diffuse redness of the skin and shedding of its outer layer
   A. 1 and 2 only
   B. 1 and 3 only
   C. 2 and 3 only
   D. 1, 2, and 3

6. Which of the following terms describes the amount of energy per unit mass transferred from an x-ray beam to an object?
   A. SI
   B. Exposure
   C. Equivalent dose
   D. Absorbed dose

7. To determine D, the amount of energy absorbed by the irradiated object must be measured by
   A. Calculating the EqD
   B. Calculating the entrance-skin exposure of the object
   C. Determining the amount of energy deposited per kilogram of the irradiated object
   D. Determining the amount of ionization in a specified volume of dry air at atmospheric pressure

8. LET is expressed in units of
   A. EfD
   B. EqD
   C. keV/μm
   D. Person-sievert

9. The EfD is based on which of the following?
   A. The energy deposited in biologic tissue by ionizing radiation
   B. The electrical charge produced in a kilogram of dry air by ionizing radiation
   C. The dose of ionizing radiation required to cause diffuse redness over an area of skin
   D. The number of electron-ion pairs in a specific volume of air

10. Which of the following is the radiation unit used for calibration of diagnostic x-ray equipment performed with an ionization chamber?
    A. Sv (rem)
    B. Gy (rad)
    C. Rem (rom)
    D. C/kg (R)

11. Which of the following radiation quantities can be used to compare the average amount of radiation received by the entire body from a specific radiologic examination with the amount received from natural background radiation?
    A. D
    B. EfD
    C. EqD
    D. Exposure

12. Which of the following radiation quantities is used to describe population or group exposure from low doses of different sources of ionizing radiation?
    A. D
    B. EqD
    C. Exposure
    D. ColEfD

13. A W_R has been established for the following ionizing radiations: x-rays ($W_R = 1$); fast neutrons ($W_R = 20$); and alpha particles ($W_R = 20$). What is the *total* EqD (in rem) for a person who has received the following exposures: x-rays = 4 rads; fast neutrons = 6 rads, and alpha particles = 3 rads?
    A. 1.84
    B. 18.4
    C. 184
    D. 1840

14. A dimensionless factor, or multiplier, that places risks associated with biologic effects on a common scale is known as the
    A. D
    B. Background time factor
    C. EqD
    D. W_R

15. Which of the following have similar numeric values?
    1. Quality factor (Q)
    2. W_R
    3. W_T
    A. 1 and 2 only
    B. 1 and 3 only
    C. 2 and 3 only
    D. 1, 2, and 3

16. If a patient undergoing x-ray therapy receives a total dosage of 3000 rads, the dosage may be recorded as _____ if the SI system is used.
    A. 6000 Gy
    B. 3000 centigray (cGy)
    C. 300 rads
    D. 30 R

17. Which of the following radiations have a W_R of 20?
    A. Alpha particles
    B. Gamma radiation
    C. Neutrons, energy <10 keV
    D. X-radiation

18. Ten Sv equals _____ rem.
    A. 10
    B. 100
    C. 1000
    D. 10,000

19. Which of the following is (are) equivalent to 1 rem?
    1. $^1/_{100}$ Sv
    2. 1 centisievert (cSv)
    3. 10 millisieverts (mSv)
    A. 1 only
    B. 2 only
    C. 3 only
    D. 1, 2, and 3

20. Thomas A. Edison invented the
    A. Cold cathode x-ray tube
    B. Hot cathode x-ray tube
    C. Fluoroscope
    D. Standard ionization chamber

21. Which of the following are not traditional units?
    A. C/kg
    B. Gy and Sv
    C. R, rad, rem
    D. A and B

22. The ampere is the SI unit of
    A. Electrical charge
    B. Electrical current
    C. Electrical resistance
    D. X-ray ionization in air

23. One rad is equivalent to an energy transfer of
    A. 500 erg per gram of irradiated object
    B. 300 erg per gram of irradiated object
    C. 200 erg per gram of irradiated object
    D. 100 erg per gram of irradiated object

24. X-rays, beta particles (high-speed electrons), and gamma rays have been given a numeric adjustment value of 1 because they produce
    A. No biologic effect in body tissue for equal absorbed doses
    B. Varying degrees of biologic effect in body tissue for equal absorbed doses
    C. High-dose biologic effects in all body tissues for even the smallest dose
    D. Virtually the same biologic effect in body tissue for equal absorbed doses

25. In therapeutic radiology, which of the following units is replacing the rad for recording of the absorbed dose?
    A. cGy
    B. Milligray (mGy)
    C. mSv
    D. Sv

Exercise 4—True or False

Circle *T* if the statement listed below is true; circle *F* if the statement is false.

1. T F Wilhelm Conrad Roentgen discovered x-rays on November 8, 1895, at the University of Wurzburg in Bavaria, Germany.

2. T F When x-rays were discovered, a charge was being passed through a pear-shaped, partial vacuum discharge tube. Light was seen emanating from a piece of paper coated with calcium tungstate that lay on a bench several feet away.

3. T F Cancer deaths among physicians attributed to x-ray exposure were reported as early as 1910.

4. T F The British X-ray and Radium Protection Committee was formed in 1921 to investi-gate methods for reducing radiation exposure because medical professionals were alarmed by the increasing number of radiation injuries reported.

5. T F By the 1950s the EfD had replaced the toler-ance dose for radiation protection purposes.

6. T F In 1991 tissue weighting factors were revised by the NCRP based on data from more recent epidemiologic studies of the Chernobyl survivors.

7. T F Fluoroscopic entrance exposure rates are measured in roentgens per minute (R/min), and essentially all radiation survey instru-ments provide readings in traditional units.

8. T F The SI unit of absorbed dose, the gray, was named after the English radiobiologist Dorian Gray.

9. T F The ampere is the SI unit of electrical current.

10. T F Sv and R are the units used in the calculation of the radiation quantities, EqD and EfD.

11. T F C/kg or R is used for measurement of the D.

12. T F In radiation therapy, the cGy is replacing the rad for recording of the D.

13. T F Each type and energy of radiation has a specific W_R.

14. T F As the intensity of x-ray exposure of an air volume increases, the number of electron-ion pairs produced decreases.

15. T F Absorbed energy is responsible for any biologic damage caused by exposure of tissues to radiation.

16. T F Skin erythema dose was an accurate means of measuring radiation exposure because the same amount of radiation produced erythema in all patients.

17. T F In 1991 the ICRP revised tissue weighting factors based on data from more recent epidemiologic studies of atomic bomb survivors.

18. T F The EfD is based on the energy deposited in biologic tissue by ionizing radiation.

19. T F The lower the atomic number of a material, the more x-ray energy it absorbs.

20. T F Radiation weighting factors are selected by national and international scientific advisory bodies (NCRP, ICRP) and are based on quality factors and LET.

21. T F The EqD for measuring biologic effects may be determined and expressed in C/kg (SI system) or in R (traditional system).

22. T F The concept of tolerance dose originally was developed to protect occupationally exposed individuals from acute affects, such as erythema of the skin.

23. T F Sv or rem is used for the D measurement.

24. T F The EfD can be expressed in Sv or mSv.

25. T F By the 1970s dosimetry and risk analysis had become quite sophisticated.

Exercise 5—Fill in the Blank

Fill in the blanks with the word or words that best complete the statements below.

1. In late November 1895, _____ _____ took the world's first x-ray picture on film, which clearly showed the bones of his wife's hand.

2. Many of the skin lesions on the hands and fingers of early radiologists and dentists eventually became _____ as a consequence of continual exposure to ionizing radiation.

3. Because the amount of radiation required to produce an _____ reaction varied from person to person, this type of reaction was a crude and inaccurate way to measure radiation exposure.

4. In 1937 the roentgen was accepted internationally as the unit of measurement for _____ to x-radiation and gamma radiation.

5. By the 1970s recognition was growing that the health consequences for the human body as a whole organism depended on which _____ and _____ _____ had been irradiated.

6. _____ _____ is the deposition of energy per unit mass by ionizing radiation in the patient's body tissue.

7. A _____ represents the amount of electrical charge flowing past a point in a circuit in 1 second when an electrical current of 1 ampere is used.

8. X-rays, beta particles (high-speed electrons), and gamma rays produce virtually the same _____ _____ in body tissue for equal absorbed doses.

9. The EqD for measuring biologic effects may be determined and expressed in _____ or in _____.

10. The W_T accounts for the _____ to the _____ organism brought on by irradiation of individual tissues and organs.

11. Rem is an acronym for _____ _____ _____.

12. Trade or government desk work is considered a (n) _____ occupation.

13. By the 1970s radiation units were developed that included factors that accounted for the varied biologic effects of _____ types of radiation.

14. In order to measure patient and personnel exposure in a consistent, uniform manner, diagnostic imaging personnel must be familiar with the standardized radiation _____ and _____.

15. In 1921 the British X-ray and Radium Protection Committee was formed to investigate methods for reducing radiation exposure. The members of the committee were unable to fulfill their responsibility because they could not agree on a _____ unit of radiation exposure.

16. The _____ was the principal guideline for occupational exposure during the 1930s.

17. In 1934 the U.S. Advisory Committee on X-Ray and Radium Protection recommended a tolerance dose equal to _____ R/day. In 1936, the committee reduced this dose to _____ R/day.

18. In 1937 the _____ was accepted internationally as the unit of measurement for exposure to x-radiation and gamma radiation; in 1962 this unit was redefined to improve accuracy and acceptability.

19. The phasing out of the tolerance dose concept for radiation protection purposes meant that no amount of radiation was considered completely _____.

20. The International Commission on Radiation Units and Measurements (ICRU) adopted _____ units for use with ionizing radiation in 1980 and urged full implementation of these units as soon as possible.

21. _____ was instrumental in developing the most important theory of radiation dosimetry.

22. _____ is best known for his method of determining the exposure rates at various points near linear radium sources (tubes).

23. Each radiation quantity has a particular unit of _____.

24. For precise measurement of radiation exposure in radiography, the total amount of _____ _____ an x-ray beam produces in a known mass of air must be determined.

25. A standard or free air ionization chamber contains a known amount of air with precisely measured _____, _____, and _____.

Exercise 6—Labeling

Label the following illustration and tables.

A. Standard or free air ionization chamber.

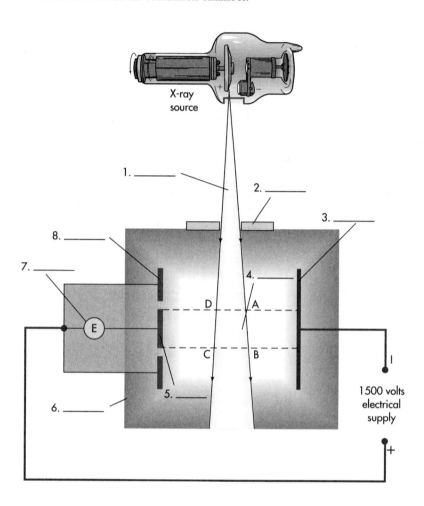

X-ray source

1. _____
2. _____
3. _____
4. _____
5. _____
6. _____
7. _____
8. _____

E

D   A

C   B

I

1500 volts electrical supply

+

B. Radiation weighting factors for different types and energies of ionizing radiation

Radiation Type and Energy Range	Radiation Weighting Factor (W$_R$)
X-ray and gamma ray photons, electrons (every energy)	1. ____
Neutrons, energy <10 keV	2. ____
10 keV to 100 keV	3. ____
>100 keV to 2 MeV	4. ____
>2 MeV to 20 MeV	5. ____
>20 MeV	6. ____
Protons	7. ____
Alpha particles	8. ____

Data adapted from International Commission on Radiological Protection (ICRP): *Recommendations, ICRP publication No. 60*, New York, 1991, Pergamon Press.

C. Summary of radiation quantities and units

Type of Radiation	Quantity	SI	Traditional Unit	Measuring Medium	Radiation Effect Measured
X-radiation or gamma radiation	1. _____	Coulomb per kilogram (C/kg)	Roentgen (R)	Air	Ionization of air
All ionizing radiations	2. _____	Gray (Gy)	Rad	Any object	Amount of energy per unit mass absorbed by object
All ionizing radiations	3. _____	Sievert (Sv)	Rem	Body tissue	Biologic effects
All ionizing radiations	4. _____	Sievert (Sv)	Rem	Body tissue	Biologic effects

Exercise 7—Short Answer

Answer the following questions by providing a short answer.

1. Why did Thomas A. Edison discontinue his x-ray research?

_____

_____

2. What unit was used for measuring radiation exposure from 1900 to 1930?

_____

_____

3. What is the difference between the short-term and the long-term somatic effects of ionizing radiation?

_____

_____

4. What is a tolerance dose?

_____

_____

5. What unit replaced the tolerance dose for radiation protection purposes in the 1950s?

_____

_____

6. In the late 1970s, dose limits were calculated and established to ensure what?

_____

_____

35

7. What is the Bragg-Gray theory and what is its significance?

_____

_____

8. When the human body is exposed to ionizing radiation, absorbed energy is responsible for what?

_____

_____

9. For a precise measurement of radiation exposure in radiography, what must be obtained?

_____

_____

10. Who is responsible for selecting radiation weighting factors and upon what are these factors based?

_____

_____

11. If the D is stated in rads, how is the Gy equivalent determined?

_____

_____

12. If the D is stated in Gy, how is the rad equivalent determined?

_____

_____

13. What unit of measure is used for calibration of x-ray equipment? Why is this unit used?

_____

_____

14. If radiation exposure is given in R, how can that value be converted to C/kg?

_____

_____

15. If radiation exposure is given in C/kg, how can that value be converted to R?

_____

_____

Exercise 8—Essay

On a separate sheet of paper, answer the following questions in essay form.

1. Describe the discovery of x-rays.

2. Discuss the impact of occupational radiation exposure on the pioneers of the radiation industry.

3. Describe the problems encountered by medical professionals as they investigated methods for reducing radiation exposure in the early 1900s.

4. Explain the changes in radiation protection criteria that led to the use of the EfD and EqD for radiation protection purposes.

5. Explain the equivalence of damage caused by radiation from different sources of ionizing radiation.

6. Explain the significance and use of a W_R.

7. Explain the significance and use of a W_T.

8. Summarize the radiation quantities and units currently in use.

9. Discuss the concept of LET and its significance.

10. Discuss the use of SI units in the field of radiology.

Exercise 9—Calculation Problems

Using the information presented below, set up and solve the following problems.

A. The SI unit of the radiation quantity, D, is the Gy; the traditional unit is the rad. Gy and rad units are easily converted to allow comparison of D values. If D is stated in rads, the equivalent Gy can be determined by dividing the rad value by 100. If D is stated in Gy, rads can be determined by multiplying the Gy value by 100.

    1. Convert 8000 rads to Gy.

    2. Convert 8 rads to Gy.

3. Convert 450 rads to Gy.

4. Convert 4.5 rads to Gy.

5. Convert 375 rads to Gy.

6. Convert 7 Gy to rads.

7. Convert 25 Gy to rads.

8. Convert 0.4 Gy to rads.

9. Convert 0.087 Gy to rads.

10. Convert 0.96 Gy to rads.

B. EqD is used for radiation protection purposes when a person receives exposure from various types of ionizing radiation. The EqD for measuring biologic effects can be determined and expressed in Sv (SI units) or rem (traditional units). The EqD is obtained by multiplying D by W_R.

1. A W_R has been established for each of the following ionizing radiations: x-radiation ($W_R = 1$); fast neutrons ($W_R = 20$); and alpha particles ($W_R = 20$). What is the total EqD in Sv for a person who has received the following exposures: x-radiation = 0.6 Gy; fast neutrons = 0.25 Gy; and alpha particles = 0.4 Gy?

2. A W_R has been established for each of the following ionizing radiations: x-radiation ($W_R = 1$); fast neutrons ($W_R = 20$); gamma rays ($W_R = 1$); protons ($W_R = 2$); and alpha particles ($W_R = 20$). What is the total EqD in Sv for a person who has received the following exposures: x-radiation = 0.3 Gy; fast neutrons = 0.28 Gy; gamma rays = 0.8 Gy; protons = 0.9 Gy; and alpha particles = 0.4 Gy?

39

3. A W_R has been established for each of the following ionizing radiations: x-radiation ($W_R = 1$); fast neutrons ($W_R = 20$); and alpha particles ($W_R = 20$). What is the total EqD in rem for a person who has received the following exposures: x-radiation = 7 rads; fast neutrons = 2 rads; and alpha particles = 5 rads?

4. A W_R has been established for each of the following ionizing radiations: x-radiation ($W_R = 1$); fast neutrons ($W_R = 20$); gamma rays ($W_R = 1$); protons ($W_R = 2$); and alpha particles ($W_R = 20$). What is the total EqD in rem for a person who has received the following exposures: x-radiation = 3 rads; fast neutrons = 0.35 rad; gamma rays = 6 rads; protons = 2.5 rads; and alpha particles = 8 rads?

5. A W_R has been established for each of the following ionizing radiations: x-radiation ($W_R = 1$); fast neutrons, energy < 10 keV ($W_R = 5$); gamma rays ($W_R = 1$); protons ($W_R = 2$); and alpha particles ($W_R = 20$). What is the total EqD in Sv for a person who has received the following exposures: x-radiation = 0.6 Gy; fast neutrons, energy < 10 keV = 0.2 Gy; gamma rays = 4 Gy; protons = 0.8 Gy; and alpha particles = 5 Gy?

C. The EfD is a quantity used for radiation protection purposes to provide a measure of the overall risk of exposure to ionizing radiation. It takes into account the dose of all types of ionizing radiation to human organs and tissues in the body that is irradiated and the overall harm (the weighting factor) of those body parts for the development of a radiation-induced malignancy (or, for the reproductive organs, the risk of genetic damage). The formula for determining the EfD is as follows: EfD = $D \times W_R \times W_T$. The EfD may be expressed in Sv (SI units) or rem (traditional units).

1. The W_R for alpha particles is 20, and the W_T for the breast is 0.05. If the breast receives a D of 0.5 Gy from exposure to alpha particles, what is the EfD in Sv?

40

2. The W_R for x-radiation is 1, and the W_T for the gonads is 0.2. If the gonads receive a D of 0.4 Gy from exposure to x-radiation, what is the EfD in Sv?

3. The W_R for fast neutrons is 20, and the W_T for the stomach is 0.12. If the stomach receives a D of 6 rads from exposure to fast neutrons, what is the EfD in rem?

4. The W_R for gamma rays is 1, and the W_T for the esophagus is 0.05. If the esophagus receives a D of 25 rads from exposure to gamma rays, what is the EfD in rem?

5. The W_R for x-radiation is 1, and the W_T for red bone marrow is 0.12. If the red bone marrow receives a D of 0.9 Gy from exposure to x-radiation, what is the EfD in Sv?

D. In addition to EqD and EfD, another dosimetric quantity, the ColEfD is used for radiation protection purposes to describe internal and external dose measurements. It is used to describe radiation exposure of a population or group arising from low doses of different sources of ionizing radiation. The ColEfD is the product of the average EfD for an individual belonging to the exposed population or group and the number of persons exposed. Therefore, ColEfD is found by multiplying the average EfD for an individual belonging to the exposed population or group by the number of individuals exposed. The radiation unit for the ColEfD is the person-sievert (the man-rem formerly was used and is obtained by multiplying the person-sievert by 100).

1. If 400 people receive an average EfD of 0.2 Sv (20 rem), what is the ColEfD in person-sievert (and man-rem)?

2. If 300 people receive an average EfD of 0.17 Sv (17 rem), what is the ColEfD in person-sievert (and man-rem)?

3. If 250 people receive an average EfD of 0.24 Sv (24 rem), what is the ColEfD in person-sievert (and man-rem)?

4. If 1000 people receive an average EfD of 0.10 Sv (10 rem), what is the ColEfD in person-sievert (and man-rem)?

5. If 100 people receive an average EfD of 0.30 Sv (30 rem), what is the ColEfD in person-sievert (and man-rem)?

POST TEST

The student should take this test after reading Chapter 3, finishing all accompanying textbook and workbook exercises, and completing any additional activities required by the course instructor. The student should complete the post test with a score of 90% or higher before advancing to the next chapter. (Each of the following 20 questions or blanks is worth 5 points.) Score = _____ %

1. If 400 people receive an average EfD of 0.2 Sv (20 rem), what is the ColEfD in person-sievert (and man-rem)?

2. Which radiation quantity can be used to compare the average amount of radiation received by the entire body from a specific radiologic examination with the amount received from natural background radiation?

_____

3. What concept helps explain the need for a radiation quality, or modifying, factor?

_____

4. In what SI unit and in what traditional unit is the radiation quantity, exposure (X), expressed?

_____

_____

5. _____ is a blood disorder that results in abnormal overproduction of white blood cells after exposure to ionizing radiation.

6. Who is credited with discovering x-rays on November 8, 1895?

_____

7. A W_R has been established for each of the following ionizing radiations: x-radiation ($W_R = 1$); fast neutrons ($W_R = 20$); and alpha particles ($W_R = 20$). What is the total EqD in Sv for a person who has received the following exposures: x-radiation = 5 Gy; fast neutrons = 0.3 Gy; and alpha particles = 0.7 Gy?

8. The W_R for x-radiation is 1, and the W_T for the lungs is 0.12. If the lungs receive a D of 2 Gy from exposure to x-radiation, what is the EfD in Sv?

9. Eight SV equals _____ rem.

10. How is the EqD calculated?

_____

11. The amount of energy per unit mass absorbed by the irradiated object is the definition of
    A. D
    B. EfD
    C. EqD
    D. X

12. The effective atomic number of bone is
    A. 7.4
    B. 7.6
    C. 13.8
    D. 20

13. _____ was used as the first measure of exposure for ionizing radiation.

14. What is the basic unit of electrical charge?

_____

15. Which of the following are short-term somatic effects of ionizing radiation?
    1. Diffuse redness of the skin
    2. Blood and intestinal disorders
    3. Nausea and vomiting
    A. 1 and 2 only
    B. 1 and 3 only
    C. 2 and 3 only
    D. 1, 2, and 3

16. One rem equals _____ mSv.

17. In radiation therapy, what SI subunit is replacing the rad for the recording of D?

_____

18. Many of the skin lesions on the hands and fingers of early radiologists and dentists eventually became _____ as a consequence of continual exposure to ionizing radiation.

19. Define the term *occupational exposure*.

_____

_____

20. On what is the EfD based?

_____

_____

4 Overview of Cell Biology

Chapter 4 covers basic concepts of cell biology. The chapter begins with a discussion of the cell and continues with other related topics, such as the chemical composition of cells. It includes a discussion of organic and inorganic compounds, cell structure, and cell division. This material lays the foundation for radiation biology, which is covered in subsequent chapters.

CHAPTER HIGHLIGHTS

- Cells are made of protoplasm, which consists of proteins, carbohydrates, lipids, nucleic acids, water, and mineral salts (electrolytes).
  - Proteins essential to growth, construction, and repair of tissue may function as hormones and antibodies.
  - Carbohydrates provide fuel for cell metabolism.
  - Lipids act as a reservoir for long-term storage of energy, guard the body against the environment, and protect organs.
  - Nucleic acids (deoxyribonucleic acid [DNA] and ribonucleic acid [RNA]) carry genetic information necessary for cell replication.
  - Water accounts for the bulk of body weight, is essential for sustaining life, and serves as the transport medium for material the cell uses and eliminates.
  - Mineral salts maintain the correct proportion of water in the cell and support cell function and conduction of nerve impulses.
- Cells have several components:
  - The cell membrane surrounds the cell, functions as a barricade, and controls passage of water and other materials into and out of the cell.
  - Cytoplasm is the portion of a cell outside the nucleus in which all metabolic activity occurs.
  - The endoplasmic reticulum (ER) transports food and molecules from one part of the cell to another.
  - The Golgi apparatus unites large carbohydrate molecules with proteins to form glycoproteins.
  - Mitochondria contain enzymes that produce energy for cellular activity.
  - Lysosomes break down unwanted large molecules; they may rupture when exposed to radiation, resulting in cell death.
  - Ribosomes synthesize the various proteins that cells require.
  - The nucleus controls cell division, multiplication, and biochemical reactions.
- Somatic cells divide through the process of mitosis.
  - The cellular life cycle has four distinct phases of mitosis: pre-DNA synthesis, actual DNA synthesis, post-DNA manufacturing, and division.
  - Mitosis has four subphases: prophase, metaphase, anaphase, and telophase.
- Genetic cells divide through meiosis.
  - Meiosis is similar to mitosis except that no DNA replication occurs in telophase; the number of chromosomes in the daughter cell is reduced to half the number of chromosomes in the parent cell.
- The Human Genome Project has mapped the entire sequence of DNA base pairs on all 46 chromosomes.
  - There are 2.9 billion base pairs arranged into about 30,000 genes.

Exercise 1—Crossword Puzzle

Use the clues to complete the crossword puzzle.

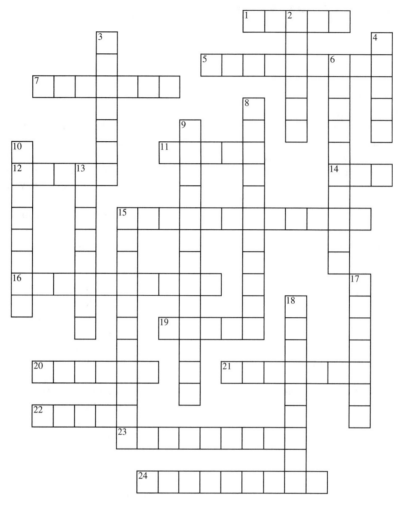

Down

2. Structural parts of cell membranes.
3. Heart of the living cell.
4. Chromosomal material.
6. Materials developed by the body in response to the presence of foreign antigens such as bacteria or viruses.
8. Tiny rod-shaped bodies.
9. Provide fuel for cell metabolism.
10. Formed by combining amino acids into long chain-like molecular complexes.
13. Small, insoluble, non-membranous particles found in the cytoplasm.
15. Coming from one zygote.
17. Process through which somatic cells divide.
18. Protein factories of the cell.

Across

1. Units of a structure that can move, grow, react, protect themselves and repair damage, regulate life processes, and reproduce.
5. Last phase of mitosis.
7. Inorganic substance.
11. Substance that aids in sustaining life.
12. The steps in the DNA ladder.
14. Female germ cells.
15. Powerhouses of the cell.
16. Unit formed from a nitrogen-containing organic base, a five-carbon sugar molecule (deoxyribose), and a phosphate molecule.
19. Inorganic substances that keep the correct proportion of water in the cell.
20. Basic constituent of all organic matter.
21. Process of reduction cell division.
22. Apparatus, or complex, that extends from the nucleus to the cell membrane and consists of tubes and a tiny sac located near the nucleus.
23. Part of the cell that lies outside the nucleus.
24. Phase of mitosis in which damage caused by radiation can be evaluated.

Exercise 2—Matching

Match the following terms with their definitions or associated phrases.

1. _____ electrolytes

2. _____ antibodies

3. _____ human genome

4. _____ cytosine and thymine

5. _____ mapping

6. _____ enzymatic proteins

7. _____ cell division

8. _____ protoplasm

9. _____ anaphase

10. _____ protein synthesis

11. _____ hormones

12. _____ genes

13. _____ sodium and potassium

14. _____ cytoplasmic organelles

15. _____ carbohydrates

16. _____ adenine and guanine

17. _____ inorganic compounds

18. _____ deoxyribose

19. _____ lipids

20. _____ protein synthesis

21. _____ interphase

22. _____ nucleic acid

23. _____ organic compounds

24. _____ lysosomes

25. _____ cell membrane

A. Chemical building material for all living things

B. Made up of a molecule of glycerin and three molecules of fatty acid

C. Controls the cell's various physiologic activities

D. Mineral salts

E. Chemical secretions manufactured by various endocrine glands

F. Process of locating and identifying genes in the genome

G. Protein production

H. Keep the correct proportion of water in the cell

I. A five-carbon sugar molecule

J. Compounds called *purines*

K. Compounds called *pyrimidines*

L. The total amount of genetic material (DNA) contained within the chromosomes of a human being

M. Protein molecules produced by specialized cells in the bone marrow called B lymphocytes

N. Multiplication process whereby one cell divides to form two or more cells

O. Saccharides

P. The phase of mitosis during which two chromatids repel each other and migrate along the mitotic spindle to opposite sides of the cell

Q. The structure that surrounds the cell and functions as a barricade to protect cellular contents from their outside environment; also controls the passage of water and other materials into and out of the cell

R. Segments of DNA that serve as the basic units of heredity

S. Small, pealike sacs or spherical bodies containing a group of digestive enzymes that are important for digestion in the cytoplasm

T. Small structures present in the cytoplasm of the cell

U. Compounds that do not contain carbon

V. All carbon compounds, both natural and artificial

W. The making of new proteins

X. Large, complex macromolecules made up of nucleotides

Y. The period of cell growth that occurs before actual cell division

Exercise 3—Multiple Choice

Select the answer that best completes the following questions or statements.

1. In human beings, how many genes are contained in all 46 chromosomes?
   A. Approximately 300
   B. Approximately 3000
   C. Approximately 30,000
   D. Approximately 300,000

2. The nucleolus contains which of the following?
   A. Centrosomes
   B. Ribonucleic acid
   C. Ribosomes
   D. Lysosomes

3. In the human cell, protein synthesis occurs in which of the following locations?
   A. Nucleus
   B. Mitochondria
   C. Ribosomes
   D. Endoplasmic reticulum

4. Interphase consists of which of the following phases?
   A. M, G_1, and S
   B. G_1, S, and G_2
   C. S, G_2, and M
   D. G_2, M, and G_1

5. Carbohydrates also may be referred to as
   A. Lipids
   B. Nucleic acids
   C. Hormones
   D. Saccharides

6. DNA regulates cellular activity *indirectly* by reproducing itself in the form of _____ to carry genetic information from the cell nucleus to ribosomes located in the cytoplasm.
   A. Messenger DNA
   B. Messenger RNA
   C. Messenger REM
   D. Transfer RNA

7. Human cells contain which four major organic compounds?
   A. Nucleic acids, water, protein, and mineral salts
   B. Mineral salts, carbohydrates, lipids, and proteins
   C. Carbohydrates, lipids, nucleic acids, and water
   D. Proteins, carbohydrates, lipids, and nucleic acids

8. Which of the following is a process of reduction cell division?
   A. Mitosis
   B. Meiosis
   C. Molecular synthesis
   D. Amniocentesis

9. Which of the following cellular organelles function as cellular garbage disposals?
   A. Endoplasmic reticulum
   B. Mitochondria
   C. Lysosomes
   D. Ribosomes

10. Which of the following describes the nuclear envelope that separates the nucleus from other parts of the cell?
    A. Single membrane
    B. Double-walled membrane
    C. Triple-walled membrane
    D. Quadruple-walled membrane

11. Which of the following are functions of the cell membrane?
    1. Protecting the contents of the cell from its environment
    2. Controlling the passage of water and other materials into and out of the cell
    3. Allowing all substances to pass
    A. 1 and 2 only
    B. 1 and 3 only
    C. 2 and 3 only
    D. 1, 2, and 3

12. Lipids are also referred to as
    A. Amino acids
    B. Carbohydrates
    C. Fats
    D. Sugars

13. The primary energy source for the cell is
    A. Amino acids
    B. Glucose
    C. Protein
    D. Phosphate

14. Cytosine bonds *only* with which of the following nitrogenous organic bases?
    A. Adenine
    B. Guanine
    C. Thymine
    D. Uracil

15. Which of the following statements is *not* true?
    A. Lysosomes are sometimes referred to as "suicide bags."
    B. Adenosine triphosphate (ATP) is essential for sustaining life.
    C. The Golgi apparatus, or complex, is the powerhouse of the cell.
    D. The nucleus is the "heart" of the cell.

16. When ionizing radiation is used to destroy malignant cells, an attempt is also made to spare healthy surrounding tissue. In radiation therapy this concept is referred to as a (an)
    A. Enzyme repair effect
    B. Therapeutic ratio
    C. Tissue tolerance effect
    D. Malignant cell annihilation effect

17. Twenty-two different _____ are involved in protein synthesis.
    A. Amino acids
    B. Antibodies
    C. Enzymes
    D. Hormones

18. The process of locating and identifying the genes in the human genome is called
    A. Gene detecting
    B. Gene extrapolation
    C. Gene tracking
    D. Mapping

19. Approximately 80% to 85% of the weight of the human body is
    A. Bone
    B. Fat-like substances
    C. Mineral salts
    D. Water

20. Meiosis is the process of
    A. Converting inorganic substances into organic substances
    B. Identifying genes in the human genome
    C. Reduction cell division
    D. Repairing breaks in DNA

21. Water performs which of the following functions in the human body?
    1. Maintains a constant core temperature of 37°C
    2. Regulates the concentration of dissolved substances
    3. Lubricates skeletal articulations (joints)
    A. 1 and 2 only
    B. 1 and 3 only
    C. 2 and 3 only
    D. 1, 2, and 3

22. Which of the following is of primary importance in maintaining adequate amounts of intracellular fluid?
    A. Deoxyribose
    B. Glucose
    C. Potassium
    D. Ribose

23. The S phase of mitosis is the
    A. Pre-DNA synthesis phase
    B. Actual DNA synthesis period
    C. Post-DNA synthesis phase
    D. Phase when DNA synthesis multiplies by a factor of 4

24. When a cell divides, the genetic-containing material contracts into tiny rod-shaped bodies called
    A. Golgi apparatus
    B. Chromosomes
    C. Mitochondria
    D. Nucleotides

25. Nitrogenous base pairs form the
    A. Hormones needed by various endocrine glands in the body
    B. Mitotic spindle
    C. Steps, or rungs, of the DNA ladderlike structure
    D. Sugars the body needs for energy

Exercise 4—True or False

Circle *T* if the statement listed below is true; circle *F* if the statement is false.

1. T F Cells are engaged in an ongoing process of obtaining energy and converting it to support their vital functions.

2. T F Depending on the cell type, water normally accounts for 25% to 35% of protoplasm.

3. T F Proper cell functioning depends on enzymes.

4. T F The skin is the body's initial barrier to any invasion by pathogens; however, once it has been penetrated, the body's primary defense mechanism against infection and disease are the hormones, which chemically attack any foreign invaders or antigens.

5. T F Lipids are organic macromolecules.

6. T F Nitrogen bonds attach the nitrogenous bases to each other, joining the two side rails of the DNA ladder.

7. T F A normal human being has 46 different chromosomes (23 pairs) in each somatic (nonreproductive) cell.

8. T F Genes control the formation of proteins in every cell through the intricate process of genetic coding.

9. T F All cellular metabolic functions occur in the nucleus.

10. T F Centrosomes are located in the center of the cell near the nucleus.

11. T F Different sequences of amino acids produce proteins with different functions.

12. T F Messenger RNA (mRNA) transfers its genetic code to another kind of RNA molecule, called *transfer RNA* (tRNA).

13. T F The cell membrane is a very thick structure that encases the human cell.

14. T F *Catabolism* is the process of breaking down organic materials to produce energy for the cell.

15. T F Water is responsible for maintaining a constant body core temperature of 37°C.

51

16. T   F   Approximately 30,000 genes are contained in all 46 human chromosomes.

17. T   F   Radiation-induced damage to chromosomes may be evaluated during telophase.

18. T   F   Water lubricates the digestive system.

19. T   F   ATP is essential for sustaining life.

20. T   F   Sodium (Na) is the primary energy source for the human cell.

21. T   F   Genes control the formation of proteins in every living cell through the intricate process of genetic coding.

22. T   F   Cells are the basic units of all living matter, but they are not essential for life.

23. T   F   Proper cell function enables the body to maintain homeostasis, or equilibrium.

24. T   F   Lipids contain the most carbon of all the organic compounds.

25. T   F   Although carbohydrates are found throughout the body, they are most abundant in the spleen and nervous tissue.

Exercise 5—Fill in the Blank

Fill in the blanks with the word or words that best complete the statement below.

1. The _____ is the fundamental component of structure, development, growth, and life processes in the human body.

2. Proper cell function enables the body to maintain _____, or equilibrium.

3. The biomolecules that compose protoplasm are formed from _____ elements.

4. Proteins are formed by combining _____ _____ into long, chainlike molecular complexes.

5. If radiation damage is excessive because of the delivered equivalent dose, the damage will be too severe for _____ _____ to have a positive effect.

6. _____ regulate body functions such as growth and development.

7. Although carbohydrates are found throughout the body, they are most abundant in the _____ and in _____ tissue.

8. The sequences of amino acids are determined by the order of the adenine-thymine and cytosine-guanine base pairs in the _____ macromolecule.

9. Maintaining the correct proportion of water in the cell maintains _____ pressure.

10. Dizygotic twins are also known as _____ twins.

11. Chromosomes are composed of _____ _____.

12. Water tends to move across cell structures or membranes into areas with a _____ concentration of ions.

13. By balancing the concentration of potassium ions (as well as sodium and chlorine ions), the cell regulates the amount of _____ it contains.

14. _____ enables the cell to perform the vital functions of synthesizing proteins and producing energy.

15. Carbohydrates provide fuel for cell _____ _____.

16. _____ synthesize the various proteins cells require.

17. Both the _____ and _____ capabilities of enzymes are vital to the survival of the cell.

18. Lipids are organic _____, large molecules built from smaller chemical structures.

19. By directing protein synthesis, the _____ _____ plays an essential role in active transport, metabolism, growth, and heredity.

20. The _____ _____ transports food and molecules from one part of the cell to another.

21. Nucleic acids (DNA, RNA) carry genetic information necessary for cell _____ _____.

22. _____ break down unwanted large molecules; they may rupture when exposed to radiation, resulting in cell death.

23. _____ metabolism is the breaking down of large molecules into smaller ones through the process of oxidation.

24. _____ are chemical compounds that result from the interaction of an acid and a base.

25. Salts are sometimes referred to as _____ _____.

Exercise 6—Labeling

Label the following illustrations and table.

A. Typical cell.

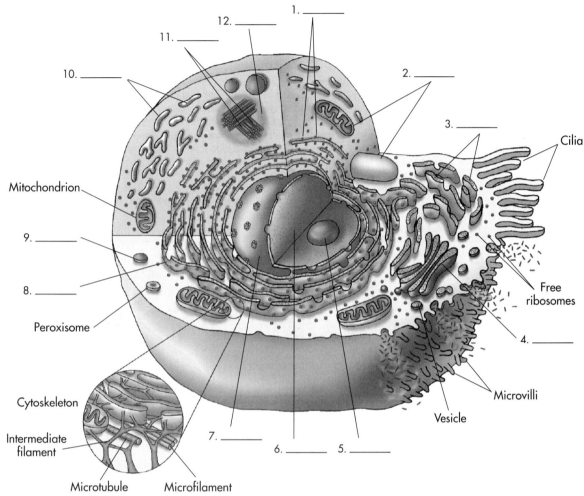

1. _____

12. _____

11. _____

10. _____

2. _____

3. _____

Cilia

Mitochondrion

9. _____

Free ribosomes

8. _____

Peroxisome

4. _____

Cytoskeleton

Microvilli

Intermediate filament

Vesicle

7. _____

6. _____   5. _____

Microtubule   Microfilament

From Thibodeau A: *Anatomy and physiology*, ed 5, St Louis, 2003, Mosby.

B. Cellular life cycle.

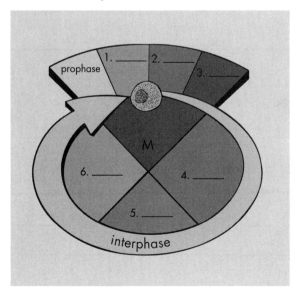

prophase

1. _____ 2. _____ 3. _____

M

6. _____ 4. _____

5. _____

interphase

From Bushong SC: *Radiologic science for technologists: physics, biology, and protection*, St Louis, ed 8, 2004, Elsevier.

C. Summary of cell components

Title	Site	Activity
1. _____	Cytoplasm	Functions as a barricade to protect cellular contents from their environment and controls the passage of water and other materials into and out of the cell; performs many additional functions such as elimination of wastes and refining of material for energy through breakdown of the materials
2. _____	Cytoplasm	Enables the cell to communicate with the extracellular environment and transfers food from one part of the cell to another
3. _____	Cytoplasm	Unites large carbohydrate molecules and combines them with proteins to form glycoproteins and transports enzymes and hormones through the cell membrane so that they can exit the cell, enter the bloodstream, and be carried to areas of the body in which they are required
4. _____	Cytoplasm	Produce energy for cellular activity by breaking down nutrients through a process of oxidation
5. _____	Cytoplasm	Dispose of large particles such as bacteria and food as well as smaller particles; also contain hydrolytic enzymes that can break down and digest proteins, certain carbohydrates, and the cell itself if the lysosome's surrounding membrane breaks
6. _____	Cytoplasm	Manufacture the various proteins that cells require
7. _____	Cytoplasm	Believed to play some part in the formation of the mitotic spindle during cell division
8. _____	Nucleus	Contains the genetic material, controls cell division and multiplication and also biochemical reactions that occur within the living cell
9. _____	Nucleus	Holds a large amount of RNA

Exercise 7—Short Answer

Answer the following questions by providing a short answer.

1. What must the human body do to ensure efficient cell operation?

_____

_____

2. What is metabolism?

_____

_____

3. How are proteins formed? What determines the precise function of each protein molecule?

_____

_____

4. What functions do enzymatic proteins perform in the human body?

_____

_____

5. Define *lipids* and list six functions they perform in the human body.

_____

_____

6. What role do ribosomes play in the manufacture of protein by a cell?

_____

_____

7. Describe the function of water inside and outside the cells in the human body.

_____

_____

8. What does the nucleus in a human cell control?

_____

_____

9. List four distinct phases of the cellular life cycle.

_____

_____

10. How are a monosaccharide, a disaccharide, and a polysaccharide different?

_____

_____

11. List the four major classes of organic compounds found in the human body.

_____

_____

12. Define *DNA*.

_____

_____

13. Where are structural proteins found in the human body? What do they provide?

_____

_____

14. What does the nucleus in a cell control?

_____

_____

15. What are hormones? What do hormones produced in the thyroid gland control?

_____

_____

Chapter **4 Overview of Cell Biology**

Exercise 8—Essay

On a separate sheet of paper, answer the following questions in essay form.

1. Describe a typical human cell and discuss cell function in the body.

2. Describe the Human Genome Project and discuss recent advances that have been achieved and challenges that remain.

3. Explain the process of mitosis.

4. Explain the significance of inorganic and organic compounds in the human body.

5. Describe the role of enzymes in the human body.

POST TEST

The student should take this test after reading Chapter 4, finishing all accompanying textbook and workbook exercises, and completing any additional activities required by the course instructor. The student should complete the post test with a score of 90% or higher before advancing to the next chapter. (Each of the following 20 questions or blanks is worth 5 points.) Score = _____ %

1. Cells are the basic units of all living _____ and are essential for life.

2. Proteins, carbohydrates, lipids, and nucleic acids are the four major classes of _____ compounds.

3. What type of enzymes can mend damaged molecules and therefore can help the cell recover from a small amount of radiation-induced damage?

_____

4. In a DNA macromolecule, adenine (A), cytosine (C), guanine (G), and thymine (T) are the four _____ organic bases.

5. Approximately 80% to 85% of the weight of the human body is _____.

6. Describe a DNA macromolecule.

_____

_____

7. What is the process of locating and identifying genes in the human genome called?

_____

8. The large, double-membrane, oval, or bean-shaped, structures that function as the powerhouses of the cell are called
   A. Endoplasmic reticulum
   B. Golgi apparatus
   C. Mitochondria
   D. Ribosomes

9. When somatic cells divide, they undergo
   A. Centrosome removal
   B. Meiosis
   C. Mitosis
   D. Nuclear collapse

10. During which subphase can radiation-induced chromosomal damage be evaluated?

_____

11. What is the function of ribosomes in the cell?

_____

12. Approximately how many genes are contained in all 46 human chromosomes?

_____

13. If exposure to ionizing radiation damages the components involved in molecular synthesis beyond repair, what will happen to the affected cells?

_____

14. Protein synthesis involves _____ different amino acids.

15. What is formed from a nitrogen-containing organic base, a five-carbon sugar molecule, and a phosphate molecule?

_____

16. What serves as a prototype for mRNA?

_____

17. The protoplasm outside the cell's nucleus is called what?

_____

18. _____ is the period of cell growth that occurs before actual mitosis.

19. _____ act as a reservoir for long-term storage of energy, guard the body against the environment, and protect organs.

20. What is the function of the cell membrane?

_____

_____

5 | Molecular and Cellular Radiation Biology

Chapter 5 covers molecular and cellular radiation biology. The science of radiation biology encompasses the sequence of events that occurs after absorption of energy from ionizing radiation, the action of the living system to compensate for the consequences of this energy assimilation, and the injury to living systems that may be produced. This chapter provides a basic knowledge of aspects of molecular and cellular radiation biology that are relevant to the subject of radiation protection. It also provides the foundation for an understanding of radiation effects on organ systems, which are discussed in Chapter 6.

CHAPTER HIGHLIGHTS

- Linear energy transfer (LET)
  - LET is the average energy deposited per unit length of track by ionizing radiation as it passes through and interacts with a medium along its path.
  - LET is expressed in units of kiloelectron volts (keV) per micron (1 micron [μm] = 10^{-6} m).
  - Low-LET radiation (x-rays and gamma rays) mainly causes indirect damage to biologic tissues, which usually can be reversed by repair enzymes.
  - High-LET radiation (alpha particles, ions of heavy nuclei, and low-energy neutrons) can cause irreparable damage to deoxyribonucleic acid (DNA) because multiple-strand breaks in DNA can occur, and these cannot be reversed by repair enzymes.
- Relative biologic effectiveness (RBE)
  - The RBE for the type of radiation used is the ratio of the dose of a reference radiation (conventionally 250 kVp x-rays) to the dose necessary to produce the same biologic reaction in a given experiment; the reaction is produced by a dose of test radiation delivered under the same conditions.
  - As the LET of radiation increases, so do the biologic effects; the RBE quantitatively describes this relative effect.
  - RBE describes the relative capabilities of radiation with differing LETs to produce a particular biologic reaction.
- Oxygen enhancement ratio (OER)
  - The OER is a comparative measure used to determine the amount of cellular injury for a species of ionizing radiation.
- Radiation-induced damage is observed on the molecular, cellular, and organic levels.
- Radiation action on the cell is either direct or indirect, depending on the site of interaction.

- Radiation action is direct when biologic damage occurs as a result of the ionization of atoms on DNA, causing them to become inactive or functionally altered.
- Radiation action is indirect when effects are produced by reactive free radicals created by the interaction of radiation with water molecules; these unstable, highly reactive free radicals can cause substantial disruption of DNA molecules, resulting in cell death.
- High-LET radiation is more likely than low-LET radiation to cause biologic damage through direct action.
- Most x-ray damage to macromolecules is the result of indirect action.
- Point mutations commonly occur with low-LET radiation and are reversible through the action of repair enzymes.
- Double-strand breaks in DNA are associated with high-LET radiation, and repair of this type of damage is not likely to occur.
- The target theory states that if cell DNA is directly or indirectly inactivated by exposure to radiation, the cell will die.
- When a cell nucleus is significantly damaged by exposure to ionizing radiation, the cell may die or may experience reproductive death, apoptosis, mitotic death, mitotic delay, interference of function, or chromosome breakage.
- The cell survival curve is used to display the radiosensitivity of a particular type of cell; this aids in the determination of the types of cancer cells that will respond to radiation therapy.
- The Bergonié-Tribondeau law states that the most pronounced radiation effects occur in cells with the least maturity and specialization, the greatest reproductive activity, and longest mitotic phases.
  - The embryo-fetus is very susceptible to radiation damage, which can cause central nervous system (CNS) anomalies, microcephaly, and mental retardation.
  - Lymphocytes are the most radiosensitive blood cells; when they are damaged, the body loses its natural ability to combat infection and becomes more susceptible to bacterial and viral antigens.
  - Human germ cells are relatively radiosensitive; temporary sterilization occurs at 2 Gy (200 rads); permanent sterilization occurs at 5 to 6 Gy (500 to 600 rads).

Exercise 1—Crossword Puzzle

Use the clues to complete the crossword puzzle.

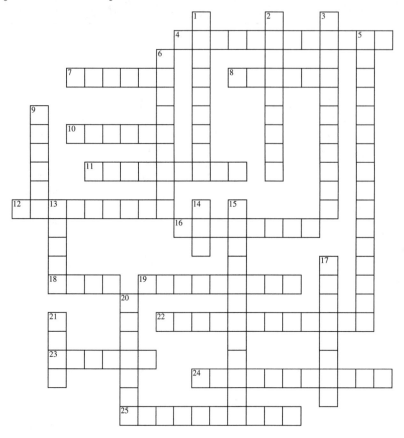

Down

1. Short-wavelength, high-energy waves emitted by the nuclei of radioactive substances.
2. Temporary condition that results from a single radiation dose of 2 Gy (200 rads) to the ovaries.
3. Process whereby single-chromosome breaks rejoin in their original configuration with no visible damage.
5. With reference to human cells and the impact of ionizing radiation upon them, this is a factor that is variable.
6. Tentacle-like extensions from a nerve cell body that carry impulses toward the cell.
9. Type of water molecule that forms when hydrogen and hydroxyl ions recombine.
13. Particle composed of two protons and two neutrons.
14. Abbreviation for important factor used in assessing potential tissue and organ damage from exposure to ionizing radiation.
15. Scavenger-type of white blood cell that fights bacteria.
17. Nonspecialized, rapidly dividing cells in the human body.
20. Type of delay that results from exposing a cell to as little as 0.01 Gy (1 rad) of ionizing radiation just before it begins dividing.
21. What an ionized atom will not be able to do properly in molecules.

Across

4. May be used to explain cell death and nonfatal cell abnormalities caused by exposure to ionizing radiation.
7. Type of tissue considered to be relatively insensitive to radiation.
8. Action that is more likely to happen after exposure to high-LET radiation.
10. Enzymes that are capable of reversing damage from a single-strand break in a DNA macromolecule.
11. A nonmitotic, or nondivision, form of cell death.
12. Blood cells that initiate clotting and prevent hemorrhage.
16. What a therapeutic dose of ionizing radiation will cause in the blood count.
18. A long, single tentacle from a nerve cell body that carries impulses toward the cell.
19. Level on which biologic damage resulting from exposure to ionizing radiation begins.
22. Small head circumference.
23. Nerve cell.
24. Cross-link formed between two places in the same DNA strand.
25. A type of breakage that is a potential outcome when ionizing radiation interacts with a DNA macromolecule.

Exercise 2—Matching

Match the following terms with their definitions or associated phrases.

1. _____ direct action

   A. Effects produced by reactive free radicals, which are created by the interaction of radiation with a water molecule

2. _____ LET

   B. The cell dies if inactivation of the master molecule occurs as a result of exposure to ionizing radiation.

3. _____ covalent cross-links

   C. A solitary atom or, most often, a combination of atoms that behaves as an extremely reactive single entity as a result of the presence of an unpaired electron

4. _____ radiation weighting factor (W_R)

   D. Used to calculate the equivalent dose to determine the ability of a dose of any kind of ionizing radiation to cause biologic damage

5. _____ mutation

   E. Loss or change of a nitrogenous base in the DNA chain

6. _____ cell survival curve

   F. Lesions that result when irradiation occurs early in interphase, *before* DNA synthesis takes place

7. _____ indirect action

   G. Describes the relative capabilities of radiation with differing LETs to produce a particular biologic reaction

8. _____ OER

   H. Chemical unions created between atoms by the single sharing of one or more pairs of electrons

9. _____ apoptosis

   I. Programmed cell death

10. _____ chromosome aberrations

    J. The radiosensitivity of cells is directly proportional to their reproductive activity and inversely proportional to their degree of differentiation.

11. _____ target theory

    K. Ratio of the radiation dose required to cause a particular biologic response of cells or organisms in an oxygen-deprived environment to the dose required to cause an identical response under normal oxygenated conditions

12. _____ RBE

    L. Method of displaying the sensitivity of a particular type of cell to radiation

13. _____ chromatid aberrations

    M. Lesions that result when irradiation of individual chromatids occurs later in interphase, *after* DNA synthesis takes place

14. _____ Bergonié-Tribondeau Law

    N. Biologic damage that occurs as a result of ionization of atoms on master, or key, molecules (e.g., DNA)

15. _____ free radical

    O. Average energy deposited per unit length of track

16. _____ mitotic delay

    P. The breaking of one or both of the sugar-phosphate chains of a DNA molecule, which can be caused by exposure of the molecule to ionizing radiation

17. _____ chromosome breakage

    Q. Branch of biology concerned with the effects of ionizing radiation on living systems

18. _____ R*

    R. Injury on the molecular level resulting from exposure to ionizing radiation

19. _____ molecular damage

    S. Female and male reproductive cells

20. _____ HO_2^*

    T. A hydrogen radical and a hydroxyl radical

21. _____ germ cells

    U. Genetic mutation in which the chromosome is not broken but the DNA within is damaged

22. _____ radiation biology

    V. A hydroperoxyl radical

23. _____ hydrogen peroxide

    W. An organic neutral free radical

24. _____ point mutation

    X. $OH^* + OH^* = H_2O_2$, a substance that is poisonous to the cell

25. _____ H* and OH*

    Y. Exposing a cell to as little as 0.01 Gy (1 rad) of ionizing radiation just before it begins dividing can result in failure of the cell to start dividing on time.

Exercise 3—Multiple Choice

Select the answer that best completes the following questions or statements.

1. Radiation damage is observed on which of the following three levels?
   A. Molecular, cellular, and inorganic
   B. Molecular, cellular, and organic
   C. Microscopic, molecular, and organic
   D. Organic, inorganic, and cellular

2. Molecular damage results in the formation of structurally
   A. Changed molecules that permit cells to continue completing normal function
   B. Changed molecules that may impair cellular function
   C. Unchanged molecules that permit cells to continue functioning normally
   D. Unchanged molecules that may impair cellular function

3. According to the target theory, if only a few non-DNA cell molecules are destroyed by radiation exposure, the cell probably will
   A. Not show any evidence of injury after irradiation
   B. Show evidence of injury after irradiation
   C. Show evidence of severe impairment after irradiation
   D. Die

4. Each cell's function is determined and defined by the structures of its constituent molecules. If these structures are altered by radiation exposure, the following may result:
   1. Disturbance of the cell's chemical balance
   2. Disturbance of cell operation
   3. Failure of the cell to perform normal tasks
   A. 1
   B. 1 and 2 only
   C. 1 and 3 only
   D. 1, 2, and 3

5. Chromosome aberrations happen when irradiation occurs
   A. Early in interphase
   B. Late in prophase
   C. At the start of metaphase
   D. At the end of telophase

6. Which of the following are examples of distorted chromosomes?
   1. Anaphase bridges
   2. Dicentric chromosomes
   3. Ring chromosomes
   A. 1 and 2 only
   B. 1 and 3 only
   C. 2 and 3 only
   D. 1, 2, and 3

7. Which of the following may be used to explain cell death and nonfatal cell abnormalities caused by exposure to radiation?
   A. Covalent cross-linking
   B. Bergonié-Tribondeau Law
   C. Programmed cell death
   D. Target theory

8. X-rays and gamma rays can be referred to as streams of particles because of a property known as
   A. LET
   B. RBE
   C. Wave-particle duality
   D. Wave-particle fragmentation

9. The random interaction of x-rays with matter produces a variety of structural changes in biologic tissue, including
   1. A single-strand break in one chromosome
   2. More than one break in the same chromosome
   3. Stickiness, or clumping together, of chromosomes
   A. 1 and 2 only
   B. 1 and 3 only
   C. 2 and 3 only
   D. 1, 2, and 3

10. Why are repair enzymes *usually* able to reverse the cellular damage generally caused by low-level ionizing radiation?
    A. Damage to DNA is sublethal.
    B. Irradiated cells are hypoxic.
    C. Only organic molecules are damaged.
    D. LET failed to occur.

11. What governs the radiation dose required to cause apoptosis?
    A. Changes in the cell protein content
    B. The phase of the cell cycle the individual cell is undergoing
    C. The radiosensitivity of the individual cell
    D. The number of cells irradiated

12. Which of the following describes the ratio of the radiation dose required to cause a particular biologic response of cells or organisms in an oxygen-deprived environment to the radiation dose required to cause an identical response under normal oxygenated conditions?
    A. OER
    B. Oxygen biologic effectiveness ratio
    C. Oxygen dose-response relationship
    D. Oxygen threshold ratio

13. Which of the following is a method of displaying the sensitivity of a particular type of cell to radiation?
    A. Cell survival curve
    B. Hypoxic cell measurement curve
    C. Radiolysis of water
    D. Radiation dose-response curve

Chapter **5** **Molecular and Cellular Radiation Biology**

14. Where in the human body are lymphocytes manufactured?
    A. Bone marrow
    B. Epithelial tissue
    C. Liver
    D. Pancreas

15. Which of the following defines the ratio of the dose of a reference radiation (conventionally 250 kVp x-rays) to the dose needed to produce the same biologic reaction in a given experiment?
    A. LET
    B. RBE
    C. W_R
    D. Low-level radiation effectiveness

16. A biologic reaction is produced by 6 Gy (600 rads) of a test radiation. It takes 36 Gy (3600 rads) of 250 kVp x-ray to produce the same biologic reaction. What is the RBE of the test radiation?
    A. 3
    B. 6
    C. 9
    D. 12

17. A hydroperoxyl radical (HO_2^-) is formed when a hydrogen free radical (H^-) combines with
    A. A hydrogen ion (H^+)
    B. A hydroxyl ion (OH^-)
    C. Molecular oxygen (O_2)
    D. Another hydrogen free radical (H^-)

18. LET is an important factor for
    A. Assessing potential tissue and organ damage from exposure to ionizing radiation
    B. Assessing the characteristics of ionizing radiation (e.g., charge, mass, and energy)
    C. Determining the OER
    D. Removing electrons from tissue exposed to ionizing radiation

19. Because high-LET radiations deposit more energy per unit length of biologic tissue traversed, they are
    A. More destructive to biologic matter than low-LET radiations
    B. Significantly less destructive to biologic matter than low-LET radiations
    C. Slightly less destructive to biologic matter than low-LET radiations
    D. Not comparable to low-LET radiations because they do not deposit any energy per unit length of biologic tissue traversed

20. Ring chromosomes, dicentric chromosomes, and anaphase bridges are examples of
    A. Normal chromosomes
    B. Chromosomes about to divide
    C. Distorted chromosomes
    D. Chromosomes that carry appropriate genetic information

Exercise 4—True or False

Circle *T* if the statement listed below is true; circle *F* if the statement is false.

1. T F The human body is a living system composed of large numbers of various types of cells, most of which cannot be damaged by radiation.

2. T F Biologic damage begins with the ionization produced by various types of radiation.

3. T F The characteristics of ionizing radiation (e.g., charge, mass, and energy) are exactly the same from one type of radiation to another.

4. T F LET is an important factor in the assessment of potential tissue and organ damage from exposure to ionizing radiation.

5. T F For radiation protection purposes, low-LET radiation is of the greatest concern when internal contamination is possible.

6. T F A positive water molecule (HOH^+) and a negative water molecule (HOH^-) are basically stable.

7. T F A few hundred centigray (cGy) (rads) can kill very sensitive cells such as lymphocytes or spermatogonia.

8. T F The embryo-fetus contains large numbers of mature, specialized cells and therefore is relatively radioresistant.

9. T F A blood count is a relatively insensitive test that is unable to indicate exposures of less than 10 cGy (10 rads).

10. T F Because the ovaries of young women are less sensitive than those of older women, a higher dose of radiation is required to cause sterility in young women.

11. T F Experimental data strongly indicate that ribonucleic acid (RNA) is the irreplaceable master, or key, molecule in the human cell.

12. T F Reproductive death generally results from exposure of cells to doses of ionizing radiation in the range of 1 to 10 Gy (100 to 1000 rads).

13. T F Ionizing radiation cannot adversely affect cell division.

14. T F Although it originally was applied only to germ cells, the Bergonié-Tribondeau Law is true for all types of cells in the human body.

15. T F LD 50/60 is more practical for human beings than LD 50/30.

16. T F If radiation damages the germ cells, the damage may be passed on to future generations in the form of genetic mutations.

63

Chapter **5 Molecular and Cellular Radiation Biology**

17. T F The presence of free radicals in tissue does not affect the amount of biologic damage that results from irradiation.

18. T F X-ray photons may interact with but do not ionize water molecules in the human body.

19. T F Because hydrogen and hydroxyl ions usually recombine to form a normal water molecule, the existence of these ions as free agents in the human body is insignificant in terms of biologic damage.

20. T F A cell survival curve is constructed from data obtained from a series of experiments.

21. T F The human body is composed of different types of cells and tissues, all of which have the same degree of radiosensitivity.

22. T F In radiotherapy the presence of oxygen is not significant in terms of radiosensitivity.

23. T F The more mature and specialized in performing functions a cell is, the more sensitive it is to radiation.

24. T F Radiation affects primarily the stem cells of the hematopoietic (blood forming) system.

25. T F The higher the radiation dose to the bone marrow, the more severe is the resulting cell depletion.

Exercise 5—Fill in the Blank

Fill in the blanks with the word or words that best complete the statements below.

1. Potentially harmful effects of ionizing radiation on living systems occur primarily at the _____ level.

2. X-ray and gamma ray photons can impart _____ to orbital electrons in atoms if the photons happen to pass near the electrons.

3. Low-LET radiation generally causes _____ _____ damage to DNA.

4. High-LET radiation includes particles with substantial _____ and _____.

5. High-LET radiation is of greatest concern when _____ contamination is possible.

6. The presence of oxygen in biologic tissues makes the damage produced by free radicals _____.

7. Approximately two thirds of all radiation-induced damage is believed ultimately to be caused by the _____ free radical (OH⁻).

8. _____ mutations could result from a single alteration along the sequence of nitrogenous bases in DNA.

9. _____ of the individual cell governs the dose required to cause apoptosis.

10. When _____ _____ interacts with cell atoms and molecules, the amount of radiation energy transferred (absorbed by the tissues) plays a major role in determining the extent of the biologic response.

11. Neutrophils, a type of white blood cell, play an important role in fighting _____ _____.

12. Thrombocytes, or _____ _____, initiate blood clotting and prevent hemorrhage.

13. _____ initially respond to radiation by increasing in number.

14. A therapeutic dose of radiation causes a _____ in the blood count.

15. Epithelial tissue has no blood vessels and regenerates through the process of _____ _____.

16. Because the body constantly regenerates epithelial tissue, the cells composing this tissue are highly _____.

17. Developing nerve cells in the embryo-fetus are more _____ than the mature nerve cells of adults.

18. Irradiation of the embryo may lead to CNS anomalies, _____, and _____ _____.

19. Because mature spermatogonia are specialized and do not divide, they are relatively _____ _____ to ionizing radiation.

20. Immature spermatogonia are unspecialized and divide rapidly, therefore these germ cells are extremely _____.

21. Nerve cells have a nucleus. If the nucleus of one of these cells is destroyed, the cell _____ and is never _____.

22. Temporary sterility usually results from a single dose of _____ Gy (_____ rads) to the ovaries.

23. Permanent sterilization occurs at _____ to _____ Gy (_____ to _____ rads).

24. The embryo-fetus, which has a large number of _____, nonspecialized

cells, is much more _____ to radiation damage than is a child or an adult.

25. A whole body radiation dose of _____ Gy (_____ rads) delivered within a few days produces a measurable hematologic depression.

Exercise 6—Labeling

Label the following illustrations and box.

A. Radiolysis of water

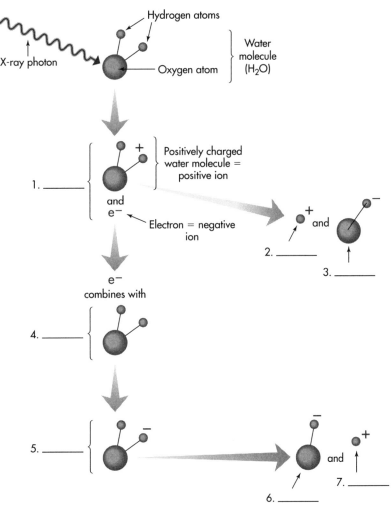

B. Indirect action of ionizing radiation on biologic molecules

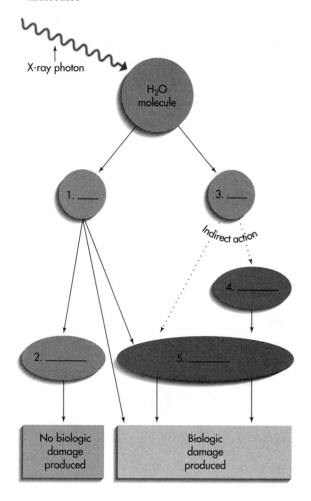

C. Examples of radiosensitivity and radioinsensitive cells

Radiosensitive Cells	Radioinsensitive Cells
1. _____	4. _____
2. _____	5. _____
3. _____	6. _____

Exercise 7—Short Answer

Answer the following questions by providing a short answer.

1. How can high-energy particles, such as alpha and beta particles and protons, ionize atoms?

_____

_____

2. What determines the extent to which different radiation modalities transfer energy into biologic tissue?

_____

_____

3. In what unit of measure is LET generally expressed?

_____

_____

4. Why can repair enzymes usually reverse the cellular damage caused by low-LET radiation?

_____

_____

5. What is a free radical?

_____

_____

6. Which cells in the human body are classified as somatic cells?

_____

_____

7. How does oxygen enhance the effects of ionizing radiation in biologic tissue?

_____

_____

8. List seven ways damage to a cell's nucleus from ionizing radiation can reveal itself.

_____

_____

9. What is the difference between direct and indirect action of ionizing radiation on atoms or molecules in the human body?

_____

_____

10. If the nucleus in an adult human nerve cell is destroyed by exposure to ionizing radiation, what will happen to the cell?

_____

_____

11. How low a dose of ionizing radiation can cause menstrual irregularities, such as delay or suppression of menstruation?

_____

_____

12. List seven possible structural changes in biologic tissue caused by the random interaction of ionizing radiation with matter.

_____

_____

13. On what three levels is radiation damage observed?

_____

_____

14. When does ionizing radiation cause complete chromosome breakage?

_____

_____

15. How was the Bergonié-Tribondeau Law established? What does it state?

_____

_____

Exercise 8—Essay

On a separate sheet of paper, answer the following questions in essay form.

1. Describe the sequence of events that can happen when an x-ray photon interacts with and ionizes a water molecule in the human body.

2. Describe the possible consequences to the embryo-fetus of exposure to ionizing radiation throughout the period of gestation.

3. Contrast the differences between high-LET radiations and low-LET radiations.

4. Discuss the cellular effects of ionizing radiation.

5. Discuss the concept of cell radiosensitivity.

POST TEST

The student should take this test after reading Chapter 5, finishing all accompanying textbook and workbook exercises, and completing any additional activities required by the course instructor. The student should complete the post test with a score of 90% or higher before advancing to the next chapter. (Each of the following 20 questions or blanks is worth 5 points.) Score = _____ %

1. A biologic reaction is produced by 7 Gy (700 rads) of a test radiation. It takes 21 Gy (2100 rads) of 250 kVp x-rays to produce the same biologic reaction. What is the RBE of the test radiation?

2. Ionizing radiation most often acts directly on which molecules in the human body to produce molecular damage through an indirect action?

_____

3. Radiosensitivity of the individual cell governs the radiation dose required to cause _____.

4. Define LET and identify how it is expressed.

_____

_____

68

5. What is a comparative measure used to determine the amount of cellular injury for a species of ionizing radiation?

_____

6. The action of ionizing radiation is _____ when biologic damage occurs as a result of the ionization of atoms on DNA, causing them to become inactive or functionally altered.

7. Because even low doses of ionizing radiation from diagnostic imaging procedures can cause chromosomal damage, which of the following should be done whenever possible?
   A. Avoid all x-ray procedures until age 60
   B. Use a low kVp and high mAs technique
   C. Shield the reproductive organs
   D. Limit all radiographic procedures to just one projection per patient

8. Immature ova are
   A. Somewhat radioinsensitive
   B. Significantly radioinsensitive
   C. Slightly radiosensitive
   D. Very radiosensitive

9. The _____ theory can be used to explain cell death and nonfatal cell abnormalities caused by exposure to radiation.

10. The action of ionizing radiation is _____ when effects are produced by reactive free radicals created by the interaction of radiation with water molecules; these unstable, highly reactive free radicals can cause substantial disruption of DNA molecules, which results in cell death.

11. What type of blood cells are classified as most radiosensitive?

_____

12. What law states that the most pronounced radiation effects occur in cells with the least maturity and specialization, the greatest reproductive activity, and the longest mitotic phases?

_____

13. Changes in genes caused by the loss of or a change in a base in the DNA chain are called _____

_____.

14. What is a cell survival curve used to display?

_____

_____

15. An ionized atom will not _____ properly in molecules.

16. What can result within a few days if an adult receives a whole body ionizing radiation dose of 0.25 Gy (25 rads)?

_____

_____

17. If bone marrow cells have not been destroyed by exposure to ionizing radiation, they can _____ _____ after a period of recovery.

18. A periodic _____ _____ is not recommended as a method of monitoring occupational radiation exposure because biologic damage already has been sustained when an irregularity is noted.

Chapter **5 Molecular and Cellular Radiation Biology**

19. During the window of maximal sensitivity, a 0.1 Sv (10 rem) fetal equivalent dose is associated with as much as a 4% risk of _____ _____.

20. When does ionizing radiation cause complete chromosome breakage?

_____

_____

6 Radiation Effects on Organ Systems

Radiation-induced damage at the cellular level may lead to measurable somatic and genetic damage throughout the living organism. Chapter 6 focuses on organic damage resulting from exposure to ionizing radiation.

CHAPTER HIGHLIGHTS

- Information obtained from a radiation dose-response curve can be used to predict the risk of malignancy in human populations exposed to low levels of ionizing radiation.
  - Curves that graphically demonstrate radiation dose-response relationships can be either linear or nonlinear and depict either a threshold or nonthreshold dose.
  - A linear nonthreshold curve currently is used for most types of cancer.
  - Risk associated with low-level radiation can be estimated with the linear quadratic nonthreshold curve.
  - Nonstochastic (deterministic) effects of significant radiation exposure may be graphically demonstrated through the use of a linear threshold curve of radiation dose-response.
  - High-dose cellular response may be demonstrated through the use of a sigmoid threshold curve.
- Acute radiation syndrome (ARS) occurs when the whole body is exposed to 6 Gy (600 rads) of ionizing radiation.
  - ARS presents in manifest as hematopoietic syndrome, gastrointestinal syndrome, or cerebrovascular syndrome.
  - ARS has four major response stages: prodromal stage, latent period, manifest illness, and recovery or death.
- Lethal dose (LD) 50/30 is used to signify the whole-body dose of ionizing radiation that can be lethal to 50% of the exposed population within 30 days.
  - The LD in humans usually is given as LD 50/60 and is estimated to be 3 to 4 Gy (300 to 400 rads).
- When cells are exposed to sublethal doses of ionizing radiation, repair and recovery are possible.
  - Surviving cells begin to repopulate.
  - Approximately 90% of radiation-induced damage may be repaired over time; 10% is irreparable.
- Early somatic effects occur within a short time after exposure to ionizing radiation.
  - Such effects include nausea, fatigue, erythema, epilation, and blood and intestinal disorders.
- Late somatic effects occur months or years after irradiation.

- Late effects include carcinogenesis, cataractogenesis, and embryologic (birth) defects.
  - Cancer is the most important late stochastic somatic effect of exposure to ionizing radiation.
  - Effects that are directly related to the dose received and that occur months or years after radiation exposure are called *late nonstochastic (deterministic) somatic effects.*
  - Effects that have no threshold, occur arbitrarily, develop independently of the dose received, and occur months or years after exposure are called *late stochastic somatic effects.*
- Risk estimates are given in terms of absolute risk or relative risk.
  - The absolute risk model predicts that a specific number of excess cancers will occur as a result of radiation exposure.
  - The relative risk model predicts that the number of excess cancers rises as the natural incidence of cancer increases in a population with age.
  - Linear and linear quadratic models are used for extrapolation of risk from high-dose data to low-dose data.
- The first trimester of pregnancy is the most critical period for radiation exposure of the embryo-fetus.
  - Radiation-induced congenital abnormalities can occur between 10 days and 6 weeks after conception.
  - Skeletal abnormalities most frequently occur between week 3 and week 20.
  - Radiation exposure in the second and third trimesters can cause congenital abnormalities, functional disorders, and a predisposition to the development of childhood cancer.
- *Genetic effects* of ionizing radiation are biologic effects on generations yet unborn.
  - Radiation-induced abnormalities are caused by unrepaired damage to deoxyribonucleic acid (DNA) within ova and sperm.
  - There is no 100% safe gonadal radiation dose; even the smallest radiation dose could cause some genetic damage.
  - The *doubling dose* measures the effectiveness of ionizing radiation in causing mutations; it is the radiation dose that causes the number of spontaneous mutations in a given generation to increase to two times their original number.
  - For human beings the doubling dose is estimated to have a mean value of 1.56 Sv (156 rem).

71

Use the clues to complete the crossword puzzle.

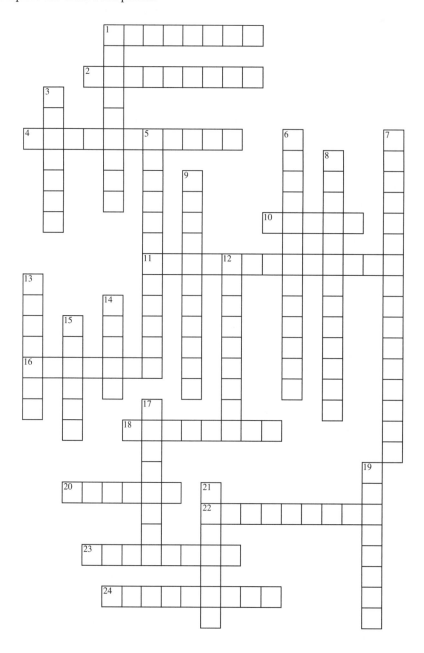

Down

1. Loss of hair.
3. Term used to describe poorly oxygenated cells.
5. Relationship that means any radiation dose will produce a biologic effect.
6. Scaling down the risk versus dose curve from high-dose data to low doses.
7. The production or origin of cataracts.
8. Period of gestation in humans which corresponds to 10 days to 6 weeks post conception.
9. Russian cleanup workers at Chernobyl.
12. All forms of life seem to be most vulnerable to radiation during this stage of development.

13. Biologic effects of ionizing radiation on future generations.
14. Project undertaken after the accident at the Chernobyl nuclear power plant to help the local population rebuild acceptable living conditions through active involvement in the reconstruction process.
15. Gland that was enlarged in many infants with respiratory distress who, in the 1940s and 1950s, eventually were treated with therapeutic doses of ionizing radiation to reduce its size.
17. The incidence of this disease in the Japanese population after detonation of the atomic bomb was

100-fold higher than normal, because many people received high doses of radiation.

19. Stage of illness in acute radiation syndrome when symptoms that were not visible in the week preceding this stage, become visible.

21. Radioactive element with a half-life of 4.5 billion years.

Across

1. Diffused redness that appears over an area of skin after irradiation.
2. Chromosomes having two centromeres.
4. Mutations that occur naturally at random and without a known cause.
10. In human beings, this is what whole-body equivalent doses of ionizing radiation greater than 12 Gy (1200 rads) are considered to be.

11. Type of studies resulting from observations and statistical analysis of data, such as incidence of disease within a group of people.

16. Type of cancer that occurred in the children of the Marshall Islanders who were inadvertently subjected to high levels of fallout during an atomic bomb test in 1954.

18. Axis of radiation dose-response curve that indicates biologic effects observed.

20. Example of a stochastic somatic effect of ionizing radiation.

22. Not considered to be a highly effective cancer-causing agent.

23. Agents that increase the frequency of occurrence of mutations.

24. Japanese atomic bomb survivors.

Exercise 2—Matching

Match the following terms with their definitions or associated phrases.

1. _____ biologic dosimetry

2. _____ probabilistic effects
3. _____ LD 50/30
4. _____ radon
5. _____ linear nonthreshold dose-response curve
6. _____ relative risk model

7. _____ bone marrow syndrome

8. _____ ETHOS Project

9. _____ linear quadratic, nonthreshold dose-response curve

10. _____ Thorotrast
11. _____ epilation

12. _____ World Health Organization

13. _____ cerebrovascular syndrome

14. _____ deterministic effects

15. _____ ARS

16. _____ absolute risk model

17. _____ doubling dose

A. Implies that the biologic response to ionizing radiation is directly proportional to the dose

B. Nonstochastic somatic effects

C. A collection of symptoms

D. Hematopoietic form of ARS

E. Stochastic somatic effects

F. Predicts that a specific number of excess cancers will occur as a result of exposure to ionizing radiation

G. A 3-year research project that began in 1996 in the Republic of Belarus in the aftermath of the accident at the Chernobyl nuclear power plant

H. Reported in 1995 that nearly 700 cases of thyroid cancer among children and adolescents were linked to the Chernobyl accident

I. Radioactive contrast agent used from 1925 to 1945 that caused liver and spleen cancer in many patients after a latent period of 15 to 20 years

J. Estimates the risk associated with low-level radiation

K. Gas that decays with a half-life of 3.8 days by way of alpha particle emission

L. Form of ARS that appears at a threshold dose of approximately 6 Gy (600 rads)

M. Whole-body dose of ionizing radiation that can be lethal to 50% of the exposed population within 30 days

N. Predicts that the number of excess cancers will increase as the natural incidence of cancer increases in a population with advancing age

O. A method of dose assessment in which biologic markers or effects of radiation exposure are measured and the dose to the organism is inferred from previously established dose-effect relationships

P. Radiation sickness that occurs in human beings after whole-body reception of large doses of ionizing radiation (1 Gy [100 rads] or more) delivered over a short time

Q. The radiation dose that causes the number of spontaneous mutations occurring in a given generation to increase to two times their original number

73

18. _____ syndrome
19. _____ prodromal stage

20. _____ gastrointestinal syndrome

21. _____ manifest illness
22. _____ embryologic effects (birth effects/defects)

23. _____ latent period

24. _____ carcinogenesis

25. _____ free radical

R. The production or origin or cancer
S. The period after the initial stage of ARS during which no visible effects or symptoms of radiation exposure occur
T. A solitary atom or, most often, a combination of atoms that behaves as an extremely reactive single entity because it has an unpaired electron
U. The stage of ARS in which symptoms become visible
V. The first stage of ARS, which occurs within hours after a whole-body absorbed dose of 1 Gy (100 rads) or more; it is characterized by nausea, vomiting, diarrhea, fatigue, and leukopenia
W. Damage to an organism that occurs as a result of exposure to ionizing radiation during the embryonic stage of development
X. Form of ARS that results when the central nervous system and the cardiovascular system receive ionizing radiation doses of 50 Gy (5000 rads) or more.
Y. Loss of hair.

Exercise 3—Multiple Choice

Select the answer that best completes the following questions or statements.

1. When biologic effects from ionizing radiation demonstrate the existence of a threshold and the severity of that damage *increases* as a consequence of increased absorbed dose, the events are considered
   A. Deterministic
   B. Probabilistic
   C. Stochastic
   D. Unimportant

2. Which of the following measures the effectiveness of ionizing radiation in causing mutations?
   A. LD 50/30
   B. Doubling dose
   C. Relative biologic effectiveness (RBE)
   D. Dose-response curve

3. Recent studies of atomic bomb survivors tend to support the _____ risk model over the _____ risk model.
   A. Absolute, relative
   B. Relative, absolute
   C. Stochastic, nonstochastic
   D. Nonstochastic, stochastic

4. The linear dose-response model is used to establish radiation protection standards because it accurately reflects the effects of
   A. Both high linear energy transfer (LET) and low-LET radiations at higher doses
   B. Both high-LET and low-LET radiations at lower doses
   C. High-LET radiations at higher doses
   D. Low-LET radiations at lower doses

5. The number of excess cancers that would *not* have occurred in a given population without exposure to ionizing radiation may be predicted by which of the following?
   1. Absolute risk model
   2. Biologic risk model
   3. Relative risk model
   A. 1 and 2 only
   B. 1 and 3 only
   C. 2 and 3 only
   D. 1, 2, and 3

6. After the accident at the Chernobyl nuclear power plant in 1986, many children in Poland and some other countries were given potassium iodide to prevent
   A. Breast cancer
   B. Bone cancer
   C. Leukemia
   D. Thyroid cancer

7. *Most* radiation-induced genetic mutations are _____.
   A. Dominant mutations
   B. Expressed in first-generation offspring
   C. Spontaneous mutations unique to radiation
   D. Recessive mutations

8. On which of the following factors does somatic or genetic radiation-induced damage depend?
   1. Extent of the body area exposed
   2. Amount of ionizing radiation to which the subject is exposed
   3. Specific parts of the body exposed
   A. 1 only
   B. 2 only
   C. 3 only
   D. 1, 2, and 3

9. When exposure to ionizing radiation causes proliferation of the white blood cells, the radiation-induced disease that occurs is
   A. Anemia
   B. Erythroleukosis
   C. Granulocytopenia
   D. Leukemia

10. Radiation can induce genetic damage by which of the following means?
    A. Interacting with somatic cells of only one parent
    B. Interacting with somatic cells of both parents
    C. Altering the essential base coding sequence of DNA
    D. None of the above; radiation cannot induce genetic damage

11. Using the doubling dose concept to measure the effectiveness of ionizing radiation at causing mutations, if 9% of the offspring in each generation are born with mutations in the absence of radiation other than background levels, administration of the doubling dose to all members of the population eventually would increase the number of mutations to
    A. 18%
    B. 36%
    C. 72%
    D. 100%

12. What do the atomic bomb survivors of Hiroshima and Nagasaki, the Marshall Islanders inadvertently subjected to high levels of fallout during an atomic bomb test in 1954, and the nuclear radiation victims of the 1986 Chernobyl disaster have in common?
    A. All were exposed to low-level ionizing radiation.
    B. All were exposed to high levels of ionizing radiation, but no group members suffered any appreciable bodily damage.
    C. All were exposed to doses of ionizing radiation sufficient to cause ARS in many group members.
    D. These groups have nothing in common.

13. For a recessive mutation to appear in an offspring
    A. Both parents must have the same genetic defect.
    B. Both parents must have only dominant genes.
    C. Neither parent needs to have a genetic defect.
    D. Only one parent must have a genetic defect.

14. Early (acute) deterministic somatic effects of ionizing radiation are *not* caused by which of the following?
    A. Doses greater than 3 Gy (300 rads)
    B. Doses greater than 6 Gy (600 rads)
    C. Doses resulting from atomic bomb detonation
    D. Doses encountered in diagnostic radiology

15. All life forms seem to be *most* vulnerable to radiation
    A. During the embryonic stage of development
    B. Immediately after birth
    C. During early childhood
    D. During adolescence

16. Which of the following are examples of stochastic effects?
    A. Nausea and vomiting
    B. Epilation and fatigue
    C. Diarrhea and leukopenia
    D. Cancer and genetic defects

17. During the embryonic stage of development:
    A. All life forms seem to be most vulnerable to radiation exposure.
    B. Only a very small percentage of life forms seem to be vulnerable to radiation exposure.
    C. A significant percentage of life forms seem to be vulnerable to radiation exposure
    D. Exposure to radiation cannot damage any life form.

18. Girls who painted watch dials with radium in some factories in New Jersey in the 1920s and 1930s eventually developed which of the following conditions as a consequence of their exposure to radiation?
    1. Osteoporosis
    2. Osteogenic sarcoma
    3. Carcinomas of the epithelial lining of the nasopharynx and paranasal sinuses
    A. 1
    B. 2
    C. 3
    D. 1, 2, and 3

19. Radium decays with a half-life of 1622 years to the radioactive element
    A. Uranium
    B. Radon
    C. Plutonium
    D. Americium

20. Mutant genes cannot properly govern the cell's normal chemical reactions or properly control the sequence of _____ in the formation of specific proteins.
    A. Amino acids
    B. Enzymes
    C. Hormones
    D. Peptic acids

21. Which of the following are mutagens?
    1. Elevated temperatures
    2. Ionizing radiation
    3. Viruses
    A. 1 and 2 only
    B. 1 and 3 only
    C. 2 and 3 only
    D. 1, 2, and 3

22. The only concrete evidence that ionizing radiation causes genetic effects comes from
    A. Human populations exposed to low radiation doses
    B. Human populations exposed to moderate radiation doses
    C. Human populations exposed to high radiation doses
    D. Extensive experiments with fruit flies and mice at high radiation doses.

23. Which of the following led to the development of the doubling dose concept?
    A. Animal studies of radiation-induced genetic effects
    B. Human studies of radiation-induced genetic effects
    C. Animal studies of radiation-induced somatic effects
    D. Human studies of radiation-induced somatic effects

24. Cataracts, leukemia, and genetic mutations are examples of
    A. Diseases that are not caused by ionizing radiation
    B. Measurable radiation-induced biologic damage
    C. Diseases caused by nonionizing radiation
    D. Radiation-induced biologic damage that cannot be measured

25. ARS is actually a collection of symptoms associated with
    A. Exposure to low-level radiation
    B. Exposure to moderate-level radiation
    C. Exposure to high-level radiation
    D. Exposure to nonionizing radiations

Exercise 4—True or False

Circle *T* if the statement listed below is true; circle *F* if the statement is false.

1. T F Cataracts, leukemia, and genetic mutations are examples of measurable radiation-induced biologic damage.

2. T F If a threshold relationship exists between a radiation dose and a biologic response, even the smallest dose of ionizing radiation will have some biologic effect on a living organism.

3. T F The Biological Effects on Ionizing Radiation (BEIR) Committee believes that the linear-quadratic, threshold curve of radiation dose-response is a more accurate reflection of stochastic somatic and genetic effects at low-dose levels from low-LET radiations.

4. T F If the effects of ionizing radiation are cell killing and directly related to the dose received, they are called *nonstochastic (deterministic) somatic effects.*

5. T F A person who has received a radiation exposure sufficient to cause radiation sickness will experience the initial stage of the syndrome within hours after the whole-body absorbed dose. After this stage, no visible symptoms occur for about 1 week.

6. T F Radiation exposure causes an increase in the number of red cells, white cells, and platelets in the circulating blood.

7. T F The LD 50/30 for adult human beings is estimated to be 8 to 9 Gy (800 to 900 rads).

8. T F The Japanese atomic bomb survivors of Hiroshima and Nagasaki are examples of a human population afflicted with ARS as a consequence of war.

9. T F Research has shown that repeat radiation injuries have a cumulative effect.

10. T F Radium watch dial painters of the 1920s and 1930s provide proof of radiation cataractogenesis.

11. T F Ionizing radiation does the greatest amount of biologic damage to the human body when a small dose of sparsely ionizing, low-LET radiation is delivered to a small or radiosensitive area of the body.

12. T F ARS actually is a collection of symptoms associated with low-level radiation exposure.

13. T F Intestinal disorders are caused by radiation damage to the sensitive epithelial tissue lining the intestines.

14. T F Conclusive proof exists that low-level ionizing radiation doses (i.e., those below 0.1 Sv [10 rem]) causes a significant increase in the risk of malignancy.

15. T F Reproductive cell damage that leads to impaired fertility is an example of a late deterministic somatic effect of ionizing radiation.

16. T F Whole-body equivalent doses greater than 1 Gy (100 rads) are considered fatal regardless of medical treatment.

17. T F The effect of low-level ionizing radiation on the embryo-fetus can only be estimated.

18. T F Some experts currently theorize that all radiation exposure levels have the potential to cause biologic damage and radiographers must use thoughtful radiation safety measures whenever human beings are exposed to radiation during diagnostic imaging procedures.

19. T F Follow-up studies of the Japanese atomic bomb survivors of Hiroshima and Nagasaki who did not die of ARS have not demonstrated late deterministic and stochastic effects of ionizing radiation.

20. T F As a result of the effects of the atomic bomb in Japan and the nuclear accident at Chernobyl, the medical community has recognized the need for a thorough understanding of ARS and appropriate medical support of victims.

21. T F The explosion at the Chernobyl nuclear power plant in 1986 blasted several tons of burning graphite, uranium dioxide fuel, and other contaminants (e.g., cesium-137, iodine-131, and plutonium-239) vertically into the atmosphere in a 3-mile high, radioactive plume of intense heat.

22. T F Repeated radiation injury does not have a cumulative effect.

23. T F Organ atrophy is the most important late somatic effect caused by exposure to ionizing radiation.

24. T F The 1989 BEIR V Report supported use of the linear-quadratic model of radiation dose-response for leukemia only.

25. T F During the 1940s and early 1950s, to reduce an enlarged thymus gland in infants, physicians treated the babies with therapeutic doses of x-radiation (1.2 to 60 Gy [120 to 6000 rads]), resulting in a substantial dose to the nearby thyroid gland; this caused thyroid nodules and carcinomas some 20 years later.

Exercise 5—Fill in the Blank

Fill in the blanks with the word or words that best complete the statements below.

1. Radiation-induced damage at the cellular level may lead to measurable _____ and _____ damage in the living system.

2. A radiation dose-response curve is either _____ or nonlinear and depicts either a _____ dose or a non-threshold dose.

3. In establishing radiation protection standards, the regulatory agencies have chosen to be conservative and use a model that might _____ _____ risk but is not expected to _____ risk.

4. Depending on the length of time from the moment of irradiation to the first appearance of symptoms of radiation damage, the effects are classified as either _____ or _____ effects.

5. Three separate dose-related syndromes occur as part of the total body syndrome: _____ syndrome, _____ syndrome, and _____ syndrome.

6. During the accident at the Chernobyl nuclear power plant in 1986, without effective physical monitoring devices, biologic criteria such as the occurrence of _____ and _____ played an important role in the identification of radiation casualties in the first 2 days after the disaster.

7. Whole-body radiation doses greater than 6 Gy (600 rads) may cause the _____ of the entire population in 30 days without medical support.

8. The risk estimate for human beings of contracting cancer from low-level radiation exposure is still _____.

9. _____ is the most important late stochastic somatic effect caused by exposure to ionizing radiation.

10. According to a recent study of 146,000 U.S. radiologic technologists, those who began working before 1940 had the greatest risk of dying of _____ cancer.

11. The mean value of the radiation doubling equivalent dose for human beings, as determined from offspring of the atomic bomb survivors of Hiroshima and Nagasaki, is _____ Sv (_____ rem).

12. The human body can incorporate radium into bone because it is chemically similar to _____.

13. Radiation dose-response curves can be used to predict the risk of _____ in human populations exposed to low levels of ionizing radiation.

14. Agents that increase the incidence of mutations are known as _____.

15. Numerous studies of Japanese female atomic bomb survivors have indicated a relative risk of breast cancer ranging from _____ to as high as _____.

16. Epidemiologic data on the Hiroshima atomic bomb survivors indicate that a linear relationship exists between radiation dose and radiation-induced _____.

77

17. Radiation actually is not a highly effective _____ agent.

18. The 1986 accident at the Chernobyl nuclear power station requires long-term _____ _____ to assess the magnitude and severity of late effects on the exposed population.

19. In the 10 years after the Chernobyl disaster, the incidence of _____ cancer increased dramatically among children living in the regions of Belarus, Ukraine, and Russia, where the heaviest radioactive _____ contamination occurred.

20. Since the Chernobyl accident, the affected population continues to work toward _____ _____ their overall quality of life.

21. According to a recent study of U.S. radiologic technologists, compared with others who started working in the 1960s or later, technologists who began working before 1940 had a slightly higher risk of dying from any type of _____.

22. The _____ of the eye contains transparent fibers that transmit light.

23. Because embryonic cells begin dividing and differentiating after conception, they are extremely _____ and therefore may easily be _____ by exposure to ionizing radiation.

24. The _____ trimester of pregnancy seems to be the most crucial period with regard to irradiation of the embryo-fetus because the embryo-fetus contains a large number of _____ cells during this period of gestation.

25. During the preimplantation period (approximately 0 to 9 days after conception), the fertilized ovum divides and forms a ball-like structure containing undifferentiated cells. If this structure is irradiated with a dose in the range of 0.05 to 0.15 Gy (5 to 15 rads), embryonic _____ occurs.

Exercise 6—Labeling

Label the following illustrations and table.

A. Hypothetical radiation dose-response curves. (Hint: The terms are included in the figure legend in the textbook.)

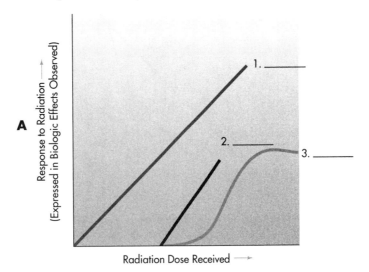

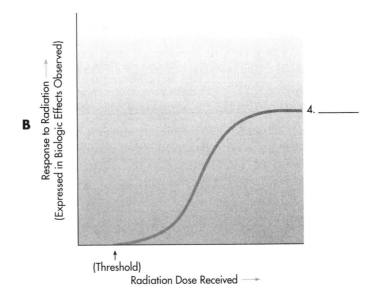

B. Hypothetical radiation dose-response curves.

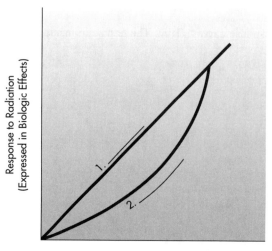

Radiation Dose

C. Overview of acute radiation lethality

Stage	Dose Gy (Rads)	Average Survival Time	Symptoms
1. ___	1 (100)	—	Nausea, vomiting, diarrhea, fatigue, leukopenia
2. ___	1–100 (100–10,000)	—	None
3. ___	1–10 (100–1000)	6 to 8 wk (doses over 2 Gy)	Nausea; vomiting; diarrhea; decrease in number of red blood cells, white blood cells, and platelets in the circulating blood; hemorrhage; infection
4. ___	6–10 (600–1000)	3–10 days	Severe nausea, vomiting, diarrhea, fever, fatigue, loss of appetite, lethargy, anemia, leukopenia, hemorrhage, infection, electrolytic imbalance, and emaciation
5. ___	5 and above (5000 and above)	Several hours to 2 or 3 days	Same as hematopoietic and gastrointestinal, excessive nervousness, confusion, lack of coordination, loss of vision, a burning sensation of the skin, loss of consciousness, disorientation, shock, periods of agitation alternating with stupor, edema, loss of equilibrium, meningitis, prostration, respiratory distress, vasculitis, coma

Exercise 7—Short Answer

Answer the following questions by providing a short answer.

1. With regard to ionizing radiation, how do threshold and nonthreshold relationships differ in terms of radiation dose and biologic response?

_____

_____

2. What type of experiments and what type of data provide the foundation for a linear, threshold curve of radiation dose-response?

_____

_____

Chapter **6** **Radiation Effects on Organ Systems**

3. Name the four stages of ARS.

_____

_____

4. Name the three forms of ARS.

_____

_____

5. According to members of the scientific and medical communities, what three categories of health effects related to low-level radiation exposure require further study?

_____

_____

6. Name three major types of late somatic effects.

_____

_____

7. What human evidence exists for radiation cataractogenesis?

_____

_____

8. What happens to fetal radiosensitivity as gestation progresses? What are the possible consequences to the developing human fetus of irradiation during the second and third trimesters of pregnancy?

_____

_____

9. What impact do mutagens such as ionizing radiation have on genetic mutations that occur as part of the natural order of events?

_____

_____

10. Name two models that researchers commonly use for extrapolation of the risk of ionizing radiation from high-dose data to low-dose data.

_____

_____

11. What evidence exists that ionizing radiation causes genetic effects?

_____

_____

12. What type of point mutations is radiation thought to cause?

_____

_____

13. What protective measures should be used routinely to minimize the possibility of genetic effects in medical imaging professionals and patients?

_____

_____

14. List the three stages of gestation in human beings and identify the time period of the pregnancy to which they correspond.

_____

_____

15. Why is LD 50/60 a more relevant indicator of outcome than LD 50/30 for human beings who have received a substantial dose of ionizing radiation?

_____

_____

Exercise 8—Essay

On a separate sheet of paper, answer the following questions in essay form.

1. Describe the mental and physical impact on the exposed population of the 1986 accident at the Chernobyl nuclear power plant.

2. Describe embryonic cell radiosensitivity during the three trimesters of pregnancy and explain radiation protection measures that must be used to protect the embryo-fetus.

3. Describe the human evidence that ionizing radiation induces cancer.

4. Explain the concept of risk as used to predict cancer incidence for populations exposed to ionizing radiation.

5. Using supportive information from Chapter 1, and information from Chapter 6, describe the ETHOS Project and explain its importance to the people in the affected areas.

POST TEST

The student should take this test after reading Chapter 6, finishing all accompanying textbook and workbook exercises, and completing any additional activities required by the course instructor. The student should complete the post test with a score of 90% or higher before advancing to the next chapter. (Each of the following 20 questions or blanks is worth 5 points.) Score = _____ %

1. What is the period of gestation in human beings that corresponds to 10 days to 6 weeks after conception?

_____

2. What is the most important late stochastic somatic effect of exposure to ionizing radiation?

_____

3. When are all life forms most vulnerable to radiation exposure?

_____

4. Using the doubling dose concept to measure the effectiveness of ionizing radiation at causing mutations, if 4% of the offspring in each generation are born with mutations in the absence of radiation other than background levels, administration of the doubling dose to all members of the population eventually would increase the number of mutations to _____ %.

5. Which risk model is used to predict that a specific number of excess cancers will occur as a result of exposure to ionizing radiation?

_____

6. What is the stage of ARS after the latent period, when symptoms become visible?

_____

7. Which radiation dose-response curve model implies that the biologic response to ionizing radiation is directly proportional to the dose?

_____

8. Revised atomic bomb data for Hiroshima and Nagasaki suggest that radiation-induced leukemias and solid tumors in the survivors may be attributed to exposure to which of the following radiations?
   A. Alpha particles
   B. Beta particles
   C. Gamma rays
   D. Neutrons

9. Which of the following groups provide evidence for radiation carcinogenesis?
      1. Radium watch dial painters (1920s and 1930s)
      2. Early medical radiation workers (1896–1910)
      3. Japanese atomic bomb survivors (1945)
   A. 1 and 2 only
   B. 1 and 3 only
   C. 2 and 3 only
   D. 1, 2, and 3

10. Define the term _nonstochastic (deterministic) somatic effects._

_____

_____

11. Where is the sigmoid, or S-shaped, (nonlinear) threshold curve of the radiation dose-response relationship generally used?

_____

_____

12. Without effective physical monitoring devices, what played an important role in the identification of radiation casualties in the first 2 days after the accident at the Chernobyl nuclear power plant?

_____

_____

Chapter **6** **Radiation Effects on Organ Systems**

13. The workers and firefighters at Chernobyl are examples of human beings who died as a result of _____ syndrome.

14. What is the estimated LD 50/30 for adult human beings if medical support is unavailable?

_____

15. How can ionizing radiation induce genetic damage?

_____

_____

16. What type of effect does repeated radiation injury have?

_____

_____

17. According to a recent study of 146,000 U.S. radiologic technologists, those who began working before 1940 had the _____ risk of dying of breast cancer.

18. With reference to ionizing radiation, what does the term *threshold* mean?

_____

_____

19. The cerebrovascular form of ARS results when the central nervous and cardiovascular systems receive doses of ionizing radiation of _____ Gy (_____ rads) or higher.

20. What currently is considered the most pronounced health consequence of the radiation accident at the Chernobyl nuclear power plant?

_____

_____

7 Dose Limits for Exposure to Ionizing Radiation

Chapter 7 discusses occupational and nonoccupational effective dose (EfD) limits and equivalent dose (EqD) limits for tissues and organs such as the lens of the eye, skin, hands, and feet. To minimize the risk of harmful biologic effects, exposure of the general public, patients, and radiation workers may be limited through adherence to established dose limits. The effective dose limiting system has been established for this purpose. This chapter also covers organizations responsible for radiation protection standards and U.S. regulatory agencies. The current radiation protection philosophy is discussed, and goals and objectives for radiation protection are identified. Other topics include the concept of as low as reasonably achievable (ALARA), the responsibilities of a radiation safety officer, the risk of radiation-induced malignancy, action limits, and the theory of radiation hormesis.

CHAPTER HIGHLIGHTS

- Effective dose limiting system
  - Adherence to occupational and nonoccupational EfD limits helps prevent harmful biologic effects of radiation exposure.
  - The concept of radiation exposure and associated risk of radiation-induced malignancy is the basis of the effective dose limiting system.
  - The sum of both external and internal whole-body exposures is considered when establishing the EfD limit.
  - Accounting for tissue weighting factors is important because various tissues and organs do not have the same degree of sensitivity.
  - Different biologic threats posed by different types of ionizing radiation must be taken into consideration even when the absorbed dose is the same.
- Effective dose limit
  - The National Council of Radiation Protection and Measurements (NCRP) has established an annual occupational EfD limit of 50 mSv (5 rem) and a lifetime EfD that does not exceed 10 times the occupationally exposed person's age in years.
  - The collective effective dose (ColEfD) describes the level of population or group exposure from low doses of different sources of ionizing radiation.
  - Internal action limits are established by health care facilities to trigger an investigation to the reasons for any unusual high exposures received by individual staff members.

- Radiation hormesis is the hypothesis that a positive effect exists for certain populations that are continuously exposed to moderate levels of radiation.
- Major organizations involved in the regulation of radiation exposure
  - The U.N. Scientific Committee on the Effects of Atomic Radiation (UNSCEAR) and the National Academy of Sciences/National Research Council Committee on the Biological Effects of Ionizing Radiation (NAS/NRC-BEIR) supply information to the International Commission on Radiological Protection (ICRP).
  - The ICRP makes recommendations on occupational and public dose limits.
  - The NCRP reviews the ICRP recommendations and incorporates them into U.S. radiation protection policy.
  - The Nuclear Regulatory Commission (NRC) is the watchdog of the nuclear energy industry; it controls the manufacture and use of radioactive substances.
  - The Environmental Protection Agency (EPA) develops and enforces regulations pertaining to the control of environmental radiation.
  - The Food and Drug Administration (FDA) regulates the design and manufacture of products used in the radiation industry.
  - The Occupational Safety and Health Administration (OSHA) monitors the workplace and regulates occupational exposure to radiation.
- Individual health care facilities establish a radiation safety committee (RSC) and designate a radiation safety officer (RSO).
  - The RSO is responsible for developing a radiation safety program for the health care facility; this person maintains personnel radiation-monitoring records and provides counseling in radiation safety.
- The ALARA concept (optimization) holds that radiation exposure should be kept as low as reasonably achievable.
- Serious radiation-induced responses may be classified as having either nonstochastic or stochastic effects.
  - *Nonstochastic effects* are biologic somatic effects of ionizing radiation that exhibit a threshold dose, below which the effect does not normally occur and above which the severity of the biologic damage increases as the dose increases.
  - *Stochastic effects* are nonthreshold, randomly occurring biologic somatic changes in which the chance of the effect occurring, rather than the severity of the effect, is proportional to the dose of ionizing radiation.

85

Exercise 1—Crossword Puzzle

Use the clues to complete the crossword puzzle.

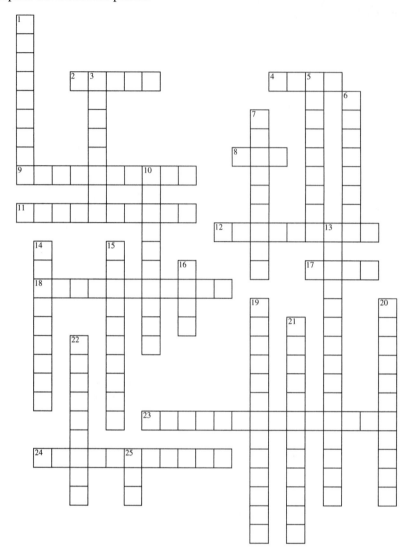

Down

1. Loss of hair.
3. The type of effective dose that must be limited to a radiation worker's age in years times 10 mSv (years × 1 rem).
5. City in Japan on which an atomic bomb was dropped.
6. Levels of ionizing radiation formerly considered acceptable by the ICRP have been revised in this direction.
7. Where OSHA regulates training programs.
10. Type of consequence of radiation for populations continuously exposed to moderately high levels of radiation that suggest a potential radiation hormesis effect.
13. What government organizations use from NCRP as the scientific basis for their radiation protection activities.
14. States in the United States that can enter into contract with the Nuclear Regulatory Commission to assume the responsibility for enforcing radiation protection regulations through their respective health departments.

15. Effects that occur random in nature and their severity is not dose dependent.
16. What the benefit obtained from any diagnostic radiologic procedure must always be weighed against.
19. Limits on radiation exposure are established by this type of Act.
20. Type of authority an RSO must have in a health care facility to stop unsafe operations.
21. Types of states in which both the state and the NRC enforce radiation protection regulations by sending agents to health care facilities.
22. What the risk of cancer induction from low absorbed doses of ionizing radiation can only be at the present time.
25. Agency established in 1970 to bring several agencies under one organization that would be responsible for protecting the health of human beings and for safeguarding the natural environment.

Across

2. As low as reasonably achievable.
4. Functions as a monitoring agency in places of employment predominantly in industry.
8. Formerly known as the Atomic Energy Commission (AEC).
9. What deterministic effects such as mental retardation are expected to be, if the equivalent dose remains below the established limit.
11. Regarding the protection of radiation workers, and the population as a whole, this is what effective dose limits have been established to serve as.
12. What the NRC writes that are presented as rules and regulations.
17. Determines the way ICRP recommendations are incorporated into United States radiation protection criteria.
18. Users of this type of material are licensed by the NRC.
23. Implementation of an effective radiation safety program in a health care facility begins with this department.
24. Irradiation of reproductive cells before conception.

Exercise 2—Matching

Match the following terms with their definitions or associated phrases.

1. _____ NCRP Report No. 116 (*Limitation of Exposure to Ionizing Radiation*)

2. _____ EfD limiting system

3. _____ EfD

4. _____ ICRP

5. _____ RSO

6. _____ UNSCEAR

7. _____ negligible individual dose (NID)

8. _____ annual occupational EfD limit

9. _____ ALARA concept

10. _____ ColEfD

11. _____ Sections 10CFR35.50 and 10CFR35.900 of the *Code of Federal Regulations*

12. _____ Annuals of ICRP

13. _____ action limits

14. _____ Radiation Control for Health and Safety Act of 1968 (Public Law 90–602)

A. Cancerous neoplasms caused by exposure to ionizing radiation

B. Optimization for radiation protection

C. Training and experience required for a RSO

D. Strictly an equipment performance standard

E. Agency that has the power to enforce radiation protection standards

F. Indicates the ratio of the risk of stochastic effects attributed to irradiation of a given organ or tissue to the total risk when the whole body is uniformly irradiated

G. Leading international organization responsible for providing clear, consistent radiation guidance through its recommendations on occupational and public dose limits

H. Lifetime EfD

I. Describes the level of radiation exposure of a population or group from low doses of different sources of ionizing radiation

J. Evaluates human and environmental ionizing radiation exposures from a variety of sources, including radioactive materials, radiation-producing machines, and radiation accidents

K. Responsible for regulations concerning employees' right to know about hazards that may be present in the workplace

L. Federal legislation requiring the establishment of minimal standards for the accreditation of educational programs for personnel who administer radiologic procedures and the certification of such individuals

M. Established by health care facilities to trigger an investigation to uncover the reasons for any unusual high exposure received by individual staff members

N. Set of numeric dose limits that are based on calculations of the various risks of cancer and genetic effects to tissues or organs exposed to radiation

87

15. _____ OSHA

16. _____ BEIR reports

17. _____ FDA

18. _____ EfD limit

19. _____ NRC

20. _____ cumulative effective dose (CumEfD) limit

21. _____ EqD limit

22. _____ tissue weighting factor (W_T)

23. _____ radiation-induced malignancy

24. _____ Consumer-Patient Radiation Health and Safety Act (Title IX of Public Law 97–35).

25. _____ Code of standards for diagnostic x-ray equipment

O. Conducts an ongoing products radiation control program, regulating the design and manufacture of electronic products, including diagnostic x-ray equipment

P. An upper boundary limit for radiation workers for yearly whole-body exposure (excluding personal medical and natural background exposure) of 50 mSv (5 rem)

Q. An annual EfD that provides a low-exposure cutoff level so that regulatory agencies may dismiss a level of individual risk as negligible

R. Normally a medical physicist, health physicist, radiologist, or other individual qualified through adequate training and experience who is designated by a health care facility and approved by the NRC and the state to ensure that a facility follows internationally accepted guidelines for radiation protection

S. Scientific journals published by the ICRP

T. A quantity that is used for radiation protection purposes to provide a measure of the overall risk of exposure to ionizing radiation. This quantity takes into account the dose for all types of ionizing radiation to organs or tissues in the human body being irradiated and the overall harm, or weighting factor, of those biologic components for developing a radiation-induced cancer (or, for the reproductive organs, the risk of genetic damage).

U. Publications that list studies of biologic effects and associated risk of groups of people who were either routinely or accidentally exposed to ionizing radiation

V. EfD recommended as an upper boundary dose of ionizing radiation that results in a negligible risk of bodily injury or genetic damage

W. Applies to complete x-ray systems and major components manufactured after August 1, 1974

X. Provides the most recent guidance on radiation protection

Y. A quantity used for radiation protection purposes that attempts to account for variation in biologic harm produced by different types of radiation. It is the product of the absorbed dose in a tissue or organ in the human body and its associated radiation weighting factor chosen for the type of radiation in question.

Exercise 3—Multiple Choice

Select the answer that best completes the following questions or statements.

1. Why have occupational and nonoccupational EfD limits been developed by scientists?
   A. To eliminate all harmful effects from low-level ionizing radiation exposure
   B. To minimize the risk of harmful biologic effects to the general public, patients, and radiation workers
   C. To promote radiation hormesis
   D. To be comparable to the risk occurring in both nonsafe and safe industries

2. Which of the following concerns the upper boundary dose of ionizing radiation that results in a *negligible risk* of bodily injury or genetic damage?
   A. Skin erythema dose
   B. Dose limits
   C. ColEfD
   D. EfD limit

3. Fundamental radiation protection standards governing occupational radiation exposure may be found in which of the following documents?
   A. 5 CFR 10
   B. 10 CFR 20
   C. *The ALARA Manual*
   D. Public Law 90–602

4. Which of the following groups are radiation protection standards organizations?
   1. ICRP
   2. NCRP
   3. UNSCEAR
   A. 1 and 2 only
   B. 1 and 3 only
   C. 2 and 3 only
   D. 1, 2, and 3

5. The NCRP recommends that radiation exposure be kept at which of the following levels?
   A. As low as reasonably achievable
   B. At threshold levels
   C. Slightly above upper boundary levels
   D. At 0.01 mSv/yr

6. Which of the following concepts is behind the establishment of the effective dose limiting system?
   A. Negligible risk
   B. Organ and tissue radiosensitivity
   C. Radiation hormesis
   D. Radiation exposure and associated risk of possible radiation-induced malignancy

7. The term *mutagenesis* refers to which of the following?
   A. Birth defects from irradiation of reproductive cells before conception
   B. Birth defects from irradiation of the unborn child in utero
   C. Cancer caused by ionizing radiation exposure
   D. Somatic effects of ionizing radiation caused by low-level exposure

8. Somatic effects of ionizing radiation that exhibit a threshold dose *below* which the effects do not normally occur and *above* which the severity of the biologic damage *increases* as the dose *increases* are classified as which of the following?
   A. Deterministic effects
   B. Epidemiologic effects
   C. Probabilistic effects
   D. Stochastic effects

9. Congress passed the Radiation Control for Health and Safety Act (Public Law 90–602) in 1968 to protect the public from the hazards of unnecessary radiation exposure resulting from which of the following?
   A. Diagnostic x-ray equipment only
   B. Therapeutic x-ray equipment only
   C. Electronic products, excluding diagnostic x-ray equipment
   D. Electronic products, including diagnostic x-ray equipment

10. Which of the following are classified as *late* deterministic somatic effects?
    1. Cataract formation
    2. Organ atrophy
    3. Radiation-induced malignancy
    A. 1 and 2 only
    B. 1 and 3 only
    C. 2 and 3 only
    D. 1, 2, and 3

11. What term is used for a *beneficial* effect of radiation in populations continuously exposed to low levels of radiation above background?
    A. Nonoccupational EqD effect
    B. Radiation negligible risk level effect
    C. Radiation hormesis effect
    D. Radiation benevolent effect

12. In addition to the annual occupational EfD limit established for radiation workers, the NCRP recommends a lifetime EfD limit, which is found by multiplying a person's age in years by which of the following?
    A. 1 mSv (0.1 rem)
    B. 10 mSv (1 rem)
    C. 100 mSv (10 rem)
    D. 1000 mSv (100 rem)

Chapter **7** **Dose Limits for Exposure to Ionizing Radiation**

13. For members of the general public not occupationally exposed, the NCRP recommends an annual EfD limit of _____ for continuous (or frequent) exposures from artificial sources of ionizing radiation other than medical irradiation and natural background and a limit of _____ annually for infrequent exposures.
    A. 1 mSv (0.1 rem), 5 mSv (0.5 rem)
    B. 3 mSv (0.3 rem), 8 mSv (0.8 rem)
    C. 10 mSv (1 rem), 20 mSv (2 rem)
    D. 50 mSv (5 rem), 75 mSv (7.5 rem)

14. Which of the following is the unit of choice for expressing the ColEfD?
    A. Group-gray (group-rad)
    B. Person-coulomb per kilogram (person-roentgen)
    C. Person-sievert (man-rem)
    D. Group-coulomb (group-roentgen)

15. A set of numeric dose limits that are based on calculations of the various risks of cancer and genetic effects to tissues or organs exposed to radiation defines
    A. ALARA concept
    B. Effective dose limiting system
    C. Investigational levels
    D. Risk protocol

16. The NRC previously was known as
    A. AEC
    B. EPA
    C. FDA
    D. OSHA

17. The Radiation Effects Research Foundation is a group run by the government of
    A. The United States to study the effects of low-level ionizing radiation on populations
    B. Germany to study the effects of ionizing radiation on the population
    C. Japan, primarily to study the atomic bomb survivors of Hiroshima and Nagasaki
    D. England to study the development of childhood cancer in children exposed in utero to ionizing radiation

18. Person-sievert (man-rem) may be used to express
    A. Annual occupational EfD for radiation workers
    B. ColEfD
    C. CumEfD
    D. EqD

19. Which agency is responsible for regulations regarding employees' right to know about hazards that may be present in the workplace?
    A. NRC
    B. All NRC agreement states
    C. EPA
    D. OSHA

20. The conclusions of the BEIR Report No. 5 about the adverse health effects of low levels of ionizing radiation are based on extrapolations from radiation EqD greater than
    A. 1 mSv (0.1 rem)
    B. 0.1 Sv (10 rem)
    C. 50 mSv (5 rem)
    D. 0.5 Sv (50 rem)

21. Because the tissue weighting factors (W_T) used to calculate EfD are so small for some organs, an organ associated with a low weighting factor may receive an unreasonably large dose even though the EfD remains within the allowable total limit. Therefore special limits are set for the crystalline lens of the eye and localized areas of the skin, hands and feet to prevent
    1. Nonstochastic effects
    2. Stochastic effects
    3. Probabilistic effects
    A. 1 only
    B. 2 only
    C. 3 only
    D. 1, 2, and 3

22. Late deterministic somatic effects (e.g., cataract formation) have a high probability of occurring when entrance radiation doses exceed
    A. 0.05 Gy (5 rads)
    B. 0.5 Gy (50 rads)
    C. 1 Gy (100 rads)
    D. 2 Gy (200 rads)

23. Established organ or tissue weighting factors for calculating the EfD include a "remainder" that takes into account additional tissues and organs, some of which are the
    1. Brain
    2. Small intestine and large intestine
    3. Uterus
    A. 1 and 2 only
    B. 1 and 3 only
    C. 2 and 3 only
    D. 1, 2, and 3

24. Using the International System (SI), the CumEfD limit to the whole body of an occupationally exposed person who is 26 years old is
    A. 26 mSv
    B. 260 mSv
    C. 2600 mSv
    D. 26,000 mSv

25. Using the traditional system, the CumEfD limit to the whole body of a 26-year-old occupationally exposed individual is
    A. 2.6 rem
    B. 26 rem
    C. 260 rem
    D. 2600 rem

Exercise 4—True or False

Circle *T* if the statement listed below is true; circle *F* if the statement is false.

1. T F The ICRP functions as an enforcement agency for radiation protection purposes.

2. T F Future radiation protection standards are expected to continue to be based on risk.

3. T F The Radiation Effects Research Foundation is a group run by the government of Japan primarily for the purpose of studying the atomic bomb survivors.

4. T F The NRC regulates and inspects x-ray imaging facilities.

5. T F In 1991 the ICRP recommended the reduction of the annual EfD limit for occupationally exposed persons from 50 mSv (5 rem) to 20 mSv (2 rem) as a result of new information obtained from the Japanese atomic bomb survivors; this information indicated that the radiation damage done by the atomic bomb detonations was approximately three to four times greater (more damaging) that previously believed.

6. T F Health care facilities that provide imaging services do not need to have an effective radiation safety program.

7. T F EfD limits may be expressed for whole-body exposure, partial-body exposure, and exposure of individual organs.

8. T F Radiation risks are derived from the complete injury caused by radiation exposure.

9. T F The Center for Devices and Radiological Health (CDRH) is responsible for credentialing radiographers.

10. T F Late deterministic somatic effects may occur months or years after high-level radiation exposure.

11. T F The ICRP is considered the international authority on the safe use of sources of ionizing radiation.

12. T F The NRC publishes rules and regulations in Title X of the *Code of Federal Regulations.*

13. T F The FDA facilitates the development and enforcement of regulations pertaining to the control of radiation in the environment.

14. T F For high-dose rate fluoroscopic procedures, entrance exposure rates as great as 20 R/min are not uncommon.

15. T F Health care facilities, such as hospitals, set their own internal action limits.

16. T F A stochastic event is an all-or-none response, meaning that ionizing radiation could cause a disease process (e.g., cancer) in the general population.

17. T F The embryo-fetus is particularly insensitive to radiation exposure.

18. T F EfD limits include radiation exposure from natural background radiation and exposure acquired when a worker undergoes medical imaging procedures.

19. T F To reduce exposure for pregnant female radiation workers and to control exposure of the unborn during potentially sensitive periods of gestation, the NCRP now recommends a monthly EqD limit to the embryo-fetus not to exceed 0.5 mSv (0.05 rem) and a limit during the entire pregnancy not to exceed 5.0 mSv (0.50 rem) after declaration of pregnancy.

20. T F In a health care facility, the RSO is meant to be a passive participant, along with the radiology department manager, in an ongoing program that prevents personnel from receiving anywhere near the maximum allowed exposures.

21. T F Lifetime survival data appear to indicate that Japanese atomic bomb survivors with moderate radiation exposure of 5 to 50 mSv (0.5 to 5 rem), the equivalent of 1.5 to 15 years of natural radiation, have a reduced cancer death rate compared with a normally exposed control population.

22. T F Employers are not required by law to evaluate their workplace for hazardous agents or to provide training and written information to their employees.

23. T F The CDRH falls under the jurisdiction of the FDA.

24. T F *Radiation hormesis* is the hypothesis that a positive effect exists for certain populations that are continuously exposed to moderate levels of radiation.

25. T F All imaging personnel should be familiar with NCRP recommendations.

Exercise 5—Fill in the Blank

Fill in the blanks with the word or words that best complete the statements below.

1. Because medical imaging professionals share the responsibility for patient safety from radiation exposure and also are subject to such exposure in the performance of their duties, they must be familiar with _____, _____, and _____ guidelines.

2. Since its inception in 1928, the ICRP has been the leading international organization responsible for providing clear and consistent radiation protection guidance through its recommendations on occupational and public _____ _____.

3. In the United States the NCRP is a _____, _____ private corporation.

4. NAS/NRC-BEIR is an advisory group that reviews studies of _____ effects of ionizing radiation and _____ assessment.

5. The EPA has the authority for determining the action level for _____.

6. The NRC licenses users of _____ materials.

7. The NRC mandates that a _____ _____ Committee be established for a facility to assist in the development of a radiation safety program.

8. Separate _____ _____ are set for occupationally exposed individuals and for the general public.

9. ALARA may also be referred to as _____ _____.

10. Cancer and genetic alterations are examples of _____ effects.

11. The limit for any education and training exposures of individuals under the age of 18 is an effective dose of _____ mSv (_____ rem) annually.

12. The ALARA concept presents an extremely conservative model with respect to the relationship between ionizing radiation and potential _____.

13. Because stochastic effects are _____, determining which members of an exposed population will develop cancer is not possible before the radiation dose is received.

14. When ionizing radiation damages reproductive cells, _____ may develop that could bring an injurious consequence in subsequent generations.

15. Currently, the risk of cancer induction from low absorbed doses of ionizing radiation can only be estimated by extrapolating (scaling down) from high-dose data, using either a _____ or _____ _____ model.

16. Revised concepts of radiation exposure and _____ have brought about recent changes in NCRP recommendations for limits on exposure to ionizing radiation.

17. The lifetime fatal risk in hazardous occupations such as logging and deep-sea fishing is many times _____ than the occupational risk associated with radiation exposure.

18. Epidemiologic studies of atomic bomb survivors exposed in utero have provided conclusive evidence of a dose-dependent increase in the incidence of severe mental retardation for fetal doses greater than approximately _____ Sv (_____ rem).

19. Referring to statement 18 above, the greatest risk for radiation-induced mental retardation occurred when the embryo-fetus was exposed ____ to ____ weeks after conception.

20. The effective dose limiting system is an attempt to equate the various risks of _____ and _____ effects to the tissues or organs that were exposed to radiation.

21. The CumEfD limit pertains to the _____ _____.

22. In addition to limits for occupationally exposed individuals, the NCRP also sets limits for _____ exposed individuals who are not undergoing medical examinations. An example of such persons would be a spouse, parent, or guardian accompanying a patient to radiology.

23. For education and training purposes, the same dose limits should apply to students of radiography in general and to those individuals under 18 years of age. The dose limit is the _____ for kindergarten thru 12th grade students attending science demonstrations involving ionizing radiation as it is for radiologic technologists under the age of 18.

24. The sum of both _____ and _____ whole-body exposures is considered when establishing effective dose limit.

25. The NCRP has established an annual occupational effective dose limit of _____ mSv (_____ rem) and a lifetime effective dose that does not exceed _____ times the occupationally exposed person's age in years.

Exercise 6—Labeling

Label the following tables.

A. Summary of radiation protection standards organizations

Organization	Function
1. _____	Evaluates information on biologic effects of radiation and provides radiation protection guidance through general recommendations on occupational and public dose limits
2. _____	Reviews regulations formulated by the ICRP and decides ways to include those recommendations into U.S. radiation protection criteria
3. _____	Evaluates human and environmental ionizing radiation exposure and derives radiation risk assessments from epidemiologic data and research conclusions; provides information to organizations such as the ICRP for evaluation
4. _____	Reviews studies of biologic effects of ionizing radiation and risk assessment and provides the information to organizations such as the ICRP for evaluation

B. Summary of U.S. regulatory agencies

Agency	Function
1. _____	Oversees the nuclear energy industry, enforces radiation protection standards, publishes its rules and regulations in Title 10 of the U.S. Code of Federal Regulations, enters into written agreements with state governments permitting the state to license and regulate the use of radioisotopes and certain other material within that state
2. _____	Enforces radiation protection regulations through their respective health departments
3. _____	Facilitates the development and enforcement of regulations pertaining to the control of radiation in the environment
4. _____	Conducts an ongoing product radiation control program, regulating the design and manufacture of electronic products, including x-ray equipment
5. _____	Functions as a monitoring agency in places of employment, predominantly in industry

C. Summary of National Council on Radiation Protection and Measurements (NCRP) Recommendations*† (NCRP Report No. 116).

A. Occupational exposures‡		
1. Effective dose limits		
a. Annual	1. __ mSv	(__ rem)
b. Cumulative	2. __ mSv × age	__ rem × age
2. Equivalent dose annual limits for tissues and organs		
a. Lens of eye	3. __ mSv	(__ rem)
b. Localized areas of the skin, hands, and feet	4. __ mSv	(__ rem)
B. Guidance for emergency occupational exposure‡ (see Section 14, NCRP #116)		
C. Public exposures (annual)		
1. Effective dose limit, continuous or frequent exposure‡	5. __ mSv	(__ rem)
2. Effective dose limit, infrequent exposure‡	6. __ mSv	(__ rem)
3. Equivalent dose limits for tissues and organs‡		
a. Lens of eye	7. __ mSv	(__ rem)
b. Localized areas of the skin, hands, and feet	8. __ mSv	(__ rem)
4. Remedial action for natural sources		
a. Effective dose (excluding radon)	9. >__ mSv	(>__ rem)
b. Exposure to radon and its decay products§	10. >__ Jhm^{-3}	(>__ WLM)
D. Education and training exposures (annual)‡		
1. Effective dose limit	11. __ mSv	(__ rem)
2. Equivalent dose limit for tissues and organs		
a. Lens of eye	12. __ mSv	(__ rem)
b. Localized areas of the skin, hands, and feet	13. __ mSv	(__ rem)
E. Embryo-fetus exposures‡		
Equivalent dose limit		
a. Monthly	14. __ mSv	(__ rem)
b. Entire gestation	15. __ mSv	(__ rem)
F. Negligible individual dose (annual)‡	16. __ mSv	(__ rem)

*Excluding medical exposures.

†See Tables 4.2 and 5.1 in NCRP Report #116 for recommendations on radiation weighting factors and tissue weighting factors, respectively.

‡Sum of external and internal exposures, excluding doses from natural sources.

§WLM stands for working level month and refers to a cumulative exposure for a working month (170 hours). As applied to radon and its daughter products, 1 WLM represents the cumulative exposure experienced in a 170-hour period resulting from a radon concentration of 100 pCi/L. The occupational limit for miners is 4 WLM per year, which results in a dose equivalent of approximately 0.15 Sv (15 rem) per year.

Exercise 7—Short Answer

Answer the following questions by providing a short answer.

1. What have scientists developed to limit radiation exposure of the general public, patients, and radiation workers?

_____

_____

2. Why must medical imaging professionals be familiar with previous, existing, and new radiation safety guidelines?

_____

_____

3. Name four major organizations responsible for evaluating the relationship between radiation EqD and induced biologic effects.

_____

_____

4. Name five U.S. regulatory agencies responsible for enforcing radiation protection standards to safeguard the general public, patients, and occupationally exposed personnel.

_____

_____

5. Why should a health care facility have a radiation safety committee?

_____

_____

6. What are the training and experience requirements for a RSO?

_____

_____

7. How do health care facilities define ALARA?

_____

_____

8. List two specific radiation protection objectives.

_____

_____

9. How is the occupational risk associated with radiation exposure equated?

_____

_____

10. Why haven't all U.S. states complied with the Consumer-Patient Radiation Health and Safety Act of 1981?

_____

_____

11. Give an example of a mutation that could cause radiation damage to reproductive cells in subsequent generations.

_____

_____

12. Give two inclusive categories that encompass the radiation-induced responses of serious concern in radiation protection programs.

_____

_____

13. What is the purpose of the Consumer-Patient Radiation Health and Safety Act of 1981?

_____

_____

14. The EPA was established for what purpose?

_____

_____

15. Define the term *exposure linearity*.

_____

_____

Exercise 8—Essay

On a separate sheet of paper, answer the following questions in essay form.

1. Discuss the current radiation protection philosophy.

2. Explain the concept of radiation hormesis.

3. Explain some of the important provisions of the code of standards for diagnostic x-ray equipment that went into effect on August 1, 1974.

4. Discuss the risk of cancer induction from high and low doses of ionizing radiation.

5. Discuss the significance of the radiation-related objectives of the NCRP.

Exercise 9—Calculation Problems

Solve the following problems.

A radiation worker's lifetime EfD must be limited to his or her age in years times 10 mSv (years × 1 rem). This is the CumEfD limit, which pertains to the whole body. Adherence to the limit ensures that the lifetime risk for these workers remains acceptable. The following problems demonstrate the application of the CumEfD limit. In the problems, EqD represents the CumEfD.

Chapter **7** **Dose Limits for Exposure to Ionizing Radiation**

1. Using the SI system, determine the CumEfD limit (in mSv) to the whole body of an occupationally exposed person who is 54 years old.

2. Using the traditional system, determine the CumEfD limit (in rem) to the whole body of an occupationally exposed person who is 54 years old.

3. Using the SI system, determine the CumEfD limit (in mSv) to the whole body of an occupationally exposed person who is 46 years old.

4. Using the traditional system, determine the CumEfD limit (in rem) to the whole body of an occupationally exposed person who is 46 years old.

5. Using the SI system, determine the CumEfD limit (in mSv) to the whole body of an occupationally exposed person who is 33 years old.

6. Using the traditional system, determine the CumEfD limit (in rem) to the whole body of an occupationally exposed person who is 33 years old.

7. Using the SI system, determine the CumEfD limit (in mSv) to the whole body of an occupationally exposed person who is 25 years old.

8. Using the traditional system, determine the CumEfD limit (in rem) to the whole body of an occupationally exposed person who is 25 years old.

9. Using the SI system, determine the CumEfD limit (in mSv) to the whole body of an occupationally exposed person who is 18 years old.

10. Using the traditional system, determine the CumEfD limit (in rem) to the whole body of an occupationally exposed person who is 18 years old.

POST TEST

The student should take this test after reading Chapter 7, finishing all accompanying textbook and workbook exercises, and completing any additional activities required by the course instructor. The student should complete the post test with a score of 90% or higher before advancing to the next chapter. (Each of the following 20 questions or blanks is worth 5 points.) Score = _____ %

1. Define risk as it relates to the radiation sciences.

_____

_____

2. The NRC is a federal agency that has the authority to control the possession, use, and production of atomic energy in the interest of _____ _____.

3. What U.S. agency functions as a monitoring agency in places of employment, predominantly in industry?

_____

4. In a health care facility, who is responsible for developing an appropriate radiation safety program to ensure that all people are adequately protected from radiation?

_____

5. Using the SI system, determine the CumEfD limit (in mSv) to the whole body of an occupationally exposed person who is 39 years old.

6. Using the traditional system, determine the CumEfD limit (in rem) to the whole body of an occupationally exposed person who is 39 years old.

7. What system is the current method for assessing radiation exposure and the associated risk of biologic damage to radiation workers and the general public?

_____

8. ALARA is the acronym for what term?

_____

9. Biologic somatic effects of ionizing radiation that can be directly related to the dose received are called
    1. Deterministic effects
    2. Stochastic effects
    3. Nonstochastic effects
  A. 1 and 2 only
  B. 1 and 3 only
  C. 2 and 3 only
  D. 1, 2, and 3

10. Examples of stochastic effects include
    1. Acute radiation syndrome
    2. Cancer
    3. Genetic alterations
  A. 1 and 2 only
  B. 1 and 3 only
  C. 2 and 3 only
  D. 1, 2, and 3

11. Currently the risk of cancer induction from low absorbed doses of ionizing radiation can only be _____ by extrapolating (scaling down) from high-dose data using either a linear or a linear quadratic model.

12. The current radiation protection philosophy is based on the assumption that a _____, _____ relationship exists between radiation dose and biologic response.

13. With what may the occupational risk associated with radiation exposure be equated?

_____

_____

14. What essential concept underlies radiation protection?

_____

_____

15. What dose limit does the NCRP recommend as an EqD limit for the embryo-fetus during the entire period of gestation?

_____

_____

16. The annual occupational EfD that applies to radiographers during routine operations is _____.

17. Why is accounting for tissue weighting factors important?

_____

_____

18. Adherence to occupational and nonoccupational _____ dose limits helps prevent harmful biologic effects of radiation exposure.

19. What is radiation hormesis?

_____

_____

20. Why are internal action limits established by health care facilities?

_____

_____

8 Protection of the Patient During Diagnostic X-Ray Procedures

Chapter 8 covers protection of the patient during diagnostic x-ray procedures. This involves limiting radiation exposure by using appropriate radiation reduction techniques, as well as protective devices that minimize such exposure. Patient exposure can be reduced substantially by the use of proper body and/or part immobilization, motion reduction techniques, appropriate beam limitation devices, adequate x-ray beam filtration, and gonadal or other specific area shielding. Selection of suitable technical exposure factors, in conjunction with either high-speed film-screen combinations or computer-generated digital images, correct radiographic film processing techniques, or appropriate digital image processing, and elimination of repeat radiographic exposures also helps to significantly limit patient radiation exposure. The chapter presents an overview of the tools and techniques used by radiographers to minimize radiation exposure to patients during diagnostic x-ray procedures.

CHAPTER HIGHLIGHTS

- Effective communication with the patient is the first step in holistic patient care.
  - Imaging procedures should be explained in simple terms.
  - Patients must have an opportunity to ask questions, and they must be given truthful answers within ethical limits.
- Adequate immobilization of the patient is necessary to eliminate voluntary motion.
  - Restraining devices are available to immobilize either the whole body or the individual body part to be radiographed.
  - Involuntary motion can be compensated for by shortening the exposure time with an appropriate increase in milliamperes (mA) and by using very-high-speed image receptors.
- X-ray beam limitation devices must be used to confine the useful beam before it enters the anatomic area of clinical interest.
  - Aperture diaphragms, cones, and extension cylinders and the light-localizing variable-aperture rectangular collimator are the beam limitation devices used.
  - The patient's skin surface should be at least 15 cm below the collimator to minimize exposure to the epidermis.
  - Good coincidence between the x-ray beam and the light-localizing beam of the collimator is necessary; both alignment and width dimensions of the two

beams must correspond to within 2% of the source-to-image receptor distance (SID).
  - According to the regulatory standard currently in effect, 2% of the SID is required with positive beam limitation (PBL) devices.
- Exposure to the patient's skin may be reduced through proper filtration of the radiographic beam.
  - Inherent filtration amounting to 0.5 mm aluminum equivalent is required.
  - Together the inherent and added filtration comprise the total filtration. Stationary x-ray units operating above 70 kVp are required to have a total filtration of 2.5 mm aluminum equivalent.
  - The beam's half-value layer (HVL) is measured to determine whether an x-ray beam is adequately filtered.
- Protective shielding may be used to reduce or eliminate radiation exposure to radiosensitive body organs and tissues.
  - The reproductive organs should be protected from exposure to the useful beam when they are in or within approximately 5 cm of a properly collimated beam unless this would compromise the diagnostic value of the study.
  - Correctly placed, appropriate gonadal shielding can greatly reduce the exposure received by both genders (50% reduction for females, 90% to 95% reduction for males).
- The clear lead shadow shield and a posteroanterior (PA) projection can significantly reduce the dose to the breast of a young patient undergoing a scoliosis examination.
- Compensating filters are used in radiography to provide uniform imaging of body parts when considerable variation in thickness or tissue composition exists.
- Appropriate technical exposure factors for each examination must be selected.
  - The techniques chosen should ensure a diagnostic image of optimal quality with the minimum patient dose.
  - Standardized technique charts should be available for each x-ray unit to help provide uniform selection of technical exposure factors. High kVp and lower mAs should be chosen whenever possible to reduce the amount of radiation received by the patient yet maintain acceptable radiographic contrast.
- Although radiographic grids increase the patient dose, their use for examination of thicker body parts is a fair

101

compromise because they remove scattered radiation emanating from the patient that otherwise would degrade the recorded image.

- □ An air gap technique can be used instead of the grid.
- Repeat radiographic exposures must be minimized to prevent the patient's skin and gonads from receiving a double dose of radiation.
- To limit the effects of inverse square falloff of radiation intensity with distance during a mobile radiographic examination, a source-to-skin distance (SSD) of at least 12 inches (30 cm) must be used.
- With digital radiography, the latent image formed by x-ray photons on a radiation detector is actually an electronic image.* The image receptor is divided into small detector elements that make up the picture elements, or pixels, of the digital image. The pixels collectively represent the information contained in a volume of tissue.†
- Radiographers must select correct technical exposure factors the first time to avoid overexposing patients when digital images are obtained.
- Computed radiography results when the invisible or latent image generated in conventional radiography is produced in a digital format using computer technology. The digital image can be displayed on a monitor for viewing and can be printed on a laser film when hard copy is needed.
- Fluoroscopic procedures produce the greatest patient radiation exposure rate in diagnostic radiology.
  - □ Patient exposure time should be minimized whenever possible.
  - □ The fluoroscopic field should be limited to the anatomic area of clinical interest.
  - □ Intermittent, or pulsed, fluoroscopy can be used to reduce the overall length of exposure.
  - □ The correct technical exposure factors should be selected to help minimize the amount of radiation received by a patient.
  - □ The x-ray SSD should be no less than 15 inches (38 cm) for stationary (fixed) fluoroscopes and no less than 12 inches (30 cm) for mobile fluoroscopes.
- During C-arm fluoroscopic procedures, the patient-image intensifier distance should be as short as possible.
- Cinefluorography can result in the highest patient doses of all diagnostic x-ray procedures.
  - □ The patient dose can be reduced by using intermittent activation of the fluoroscope to locate the catheter, limiting the time of the cine run, and using the last-hold feature to view the most recent image.
- HLC fluoroscopy is used for interventional procedures.
  - □ This operating mode uses exposure rates that are substantially higher than those allowed for routine fluoroscopic procedures.
  - □ If the skin dose is received in the range of 1 to 2 Gy (100 to 200 rads), the U.S. Food and Drug Administration (FDA) requires that a notation be placed in the patient's record.
- The amount of radiation a patient receives from diagnostic radiologic procedures may be specified as entrance skin exposure (ESE), skin dose, gonadal dose, or bone marrow dose.
  - □ ESE is the easiest to obtain and most widely used designation.
  - □ The estimated genetically significant dose (GSD) for the U.S. population is about 0.2 mSv (20 mrem).
- Nonpalpable breast cancer may be detected through mammography.
  - □ Federal regulations state that the mean dose to the glandular tissue of a 4.5 cm compressed breast using a screen-film mammography system should not exceed 3 mGy (300 mrads) per view.
- Computed tomography (CT) scanning is considered a relatively high radiation exposure diagnostic procedure because of the increasing use of multislice spiral (helical) CT scanners that use small slice thickness.
  - □ Skin dose and dose distribution are two concerns.
  - □ In spiral CT, the patient dose is comparable to that of conventional CT when the pitch ratio is about one; the patient dose is reduced when the pitch is higher and increased when the pitch is lower.
- Children are much more vulnerable to both the late somatic and genetic effects of ionizing radiation than are adults.
  - □ A PA projection should be used to protect the breasts of female patients.
  - □ When shielding is necessary in small girls, shielding of the ovaries requires shielding of the iliac wings as well as the sacral area.
  - □ Adequate collimation of the radiographic beam to include only the area of clinical interest is essential.
- A developing embryo-fetus is especially sensitive to ionizing radiation exposure.
  - □ The smallest technical exposure factors that will generate a diagnostically useful radiographic image should be used; the beam should be collimated carefully to include only the anatomic area of interest; and the lower abdomen and pelvic region should be covered with a suitable contact shield if it does not need to be included in the examination.
  - □ A radiologic physicist should determine the fetal dose if a pregnant patient is irradiated inadvertently.

---

*Bushong SC: *Radiologic science for technologists: physics, biology, and protection,* ed 8, p. 589, St. Louis, 2004, Mosby.

†Seeram E: Digital image processing, *Radiol Technol* 75:6, 2004.

Exercise 1—Crossword Puzzle

Use the clues to complete the crossword puzzle.

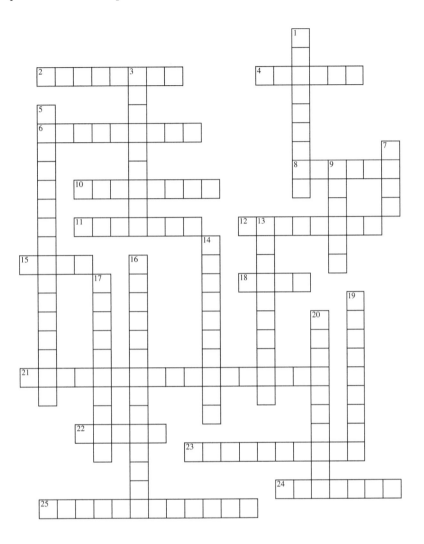

Down

1. When there is a lack of control, this type of motion results.
3. Person who should perform the calculations necessary to determine fetal exposure, if a pregnant patient is inadvertently irradiated.
5. Procedures that can result in the highest patient doses of all diagnostic procedures.
7. X-rays emitted from parts of the tube other than the focal spot.
9. Miniature square boxes in the image matrix of a digital image.

13. Radiation that scatters from the CT slice being scanned into adjacent slices.
14. Filtration material used in mammography.
16. What is needed to eliminate or at least minimize patient motion.
17. Most versatile device for defining the size and shape of the radiographic beam.
19. Scientific term referring to the brightness of a surface.
20. Placed in the path of the x-ray beam to reduce exposure to the patient's skin and superficial tissues by absorbing most of the lower energy photons from the heterogeneous beam.

Chapter **8** **Protection of the Patient During Diagnostic X-Ray Procedures**

Across

2. Rod vision, or night vision.
4. Type of fluoroscopy that involves manual or automatic periodic activation of the fluoroscopic tube by the fluoroscopist rather than lengthy continuous activation.
6. Quantity, or amount, of radiation.
8. Any radiograph that must be performed more than once because of human or mechanical error during the production of the initial radiograph thereby resulting in increased patient dose.
10. During a diagnostic x-ray procedure, this is the type of approach that is essential to patient care.
11. Type of radiation that is reduced by the use of x-ray beam limitation devices.
12. Type of cassette used for computed radiography.
15. Use of this device increases patient dose.
18. Radiation-absorbent material used to make protective shielding.
21. Dosimeters that are the sensing devices most often used to measure skin dose directly.
22. Combination of inherent plus added filtration.
23. Type of timer that must be provided and used with each fluoroscopic unit.
24. Type of shielding used to protect male and female reproductive organs during a radiographic exposure.
25. Type of filter used for dose reduction and uniform radiographic imaging of body parts that vary considerably in thickness or tissue composition.

Exercise 2—Matching

Match the following terms with their definitions or associated phrases.

1. _____ inherent filtration
2. _____ HVL
3. _____ air gap technique
4. _____ spacer bars
5. _____ added filtration
6. _____ gonadal shielding
7. _____ scattered radiation
8. _____ PBL
9. _____ computed radiography (CR)
10. _____ shaped contact shield
11. _____ high-level-control fluoroscopy (HLCF)
12. _____ carbon fiber
13. _____ gonadal dose
14. _____ effective communication
15. _____ quantum mottle
16. _____ quality control program
17. _____ off-focus radiation
18. _____ last-image-hold
19. _____ ESE

A. Standardization of film processing techniques, including monitoring and maintenance of all processors in a facility
B. Hangs over the area of clinical interest to cast a shadow in the primary beam over the patient's reproductive organs
C. Front material in a cassette that can result in a lower radiation dose for the patient because a lower radiographic technique is used to produce the recorded image
D. Device that increases the patient dose
E. Cup-shaped radiopaque device that encloses the scrotum and penis to protect the male reproductive organs from exposure to ionizing radiation
F. Feature of a radiographic collimator that automatically adjusts the collimator so that the radiation field size matches the film size
G. Allows the fluoroscopist to see the most recent image without exposing the patient to another pulse of radiation
H. An interaction that produces a satisfying result through an exchange of information
I. Thickness of a designated absorber (customarily a metal, such as aluminum) required to reduce the intensity (quantity or amount) of the primary beam by 50% of its initial value
J. Projects down from the x-ray tube housing to prevent the collimator from moving closer than 15 cm to the patient
K. Sheets of aluminum (or its equivalent) of appropriate thickness localized outside the glass window of the x-ray tube housing above the collimator shutters
L. Alternative to using a radiographic grid to reduce scattered radiation during certain examinations
M. The distance from the anode focal spot to the radiographic image receptor
N. The glass envelope encasing the x-ray tube, the insulating oil surrounding the tube, and the glass window in the tube housing
O. Devices used during diagnostic x-ray procedures to protect the reproductive organs from exposure to the useful beam while they are in or within approximately 5 cm of a properly collimated beam
P. Process in which the invisible, or latent image, generated in conventional radiography is produced in a digital format using computer technology; the digital image can be displayed on a monitor for viewing or printed on a laser film when hard copy is needed
Q. Quantity of radiation incident upon an object; backscatter is excluded
R. Image produced by computer representation of anatomic information
S. Radiation exposure received by the male and female reproductive organs

20. _____ source-to-image receptor distance (SID)

T. X-rays emitted from parts of the tube other than the focal spot

21. _____ genetically significant dose (GSD)

U. An operating mode of fluoroscopic equipment in which exposure rates are significantly higher than normally allowed for routine fluoroscopic procedures; this allows visualization of smaller and lower contrast objects than normally are visible during fluoroscopy

22. _____ radiographic grid

V. The equivalent dose to the reproductive organs that, if received by every human being, would be expected to cause an identical gross genetic injury to the total population as does the sum of the actual doses received by exposed individual population members

23. _____ useful beam

W. Faint blotches in the radiographic image produced by an intrinsic fluctuation in the incident photon intensity

24. _____ shadow shield

X. Radiation that emerges directly from the x-ray tube collimator and moves without deflection toward a wall, door, viewing window, and so on

25. _____ digital image

Y. All the radiation that arises from the interactions of an x-ray beam with the atoms of an object in the path of the beam

Exercise 3—Multiple Choice

Select the answer that best completes the following questions or statements.

1. Effective communication between the radiographer and the patient depends on which of the following?
   1. Verbal and nonverbal messages are congruent, so that they are understood as intended.
   2. The imaging procedure is explained in simple terms, and instructions are given clearly and concisely.
   3. The patient is given the opportunity to ask questions, which are answered truthfully within ethical limits.
   A. 1 only
   B. 2 only
   C. 3 only
   D. 1, 2, and 3

2. Interslice scatter during a CT scanning procedure results in which of the following?
   A. Decrease in patient dose
   B. Increase in patient dose
   C. Poorly defined cross-sectional image of the anatomy of interest
   D. Uniform distribution of radiation into all adjacent areas

3. The luminance of the collimator light source must be
   A. Adequate to outline the margins of the radiographic beam on the patient's anatomy
   B. Visible on the patient's anatomy only when all white light is turned off in the radiography room
   C. Less than 5 foot-candles
   D. At least 10 foot-candles

4. Which of the following results in an *increase* in the patient dose?
   A. Use of a radiographic grid
   B. Use of the correct radiographic processing technique
   C. Use of rare-earth intensifying screens with matching radiographic film
   D. Use of the highest practicable kVp with the lowest possible mAs for each examination

5. The patient dose *decreases* and the life of the fluoroscopic tube *increases* with which of the following?
   A. Restriction of the fluoroscopic field to include only the area of clinical interest
   B. Use of a conventional fluoroscope rather than image intensification
   C. Intermittent, or pulsed, fluoroscopy
   D. Darkness adaptation

6. An optimal quality cross-table lateral projection of the cervical spine was obtained using appropriate technical exposure factors and an 8:1 ratio grid. If another radiograph is obtained using an air gap technique and technical exposure factors that are comparable to those used with the 8:1 ratio grid, the patient dose is
   A. About the same
   B. Significantly higher
   C. Significantly lower
   D. Not an issue because an air gap technique cannot be used in place of a grid for a lateral projection of the cervical spine

7. The skin and gonads of the patient receive a "double dose" of x-radiation
   A. During all CT procedures
   B. Whenever inherent and added filtration are used during a radiographic examination
   C. Whenever high-speed screen-film image receptor systems are used
   D. Whenever a repeat radiograph occurs as a consequence of human or mechanical error

105

8. The benefits of a repeat analysis program include
    1. Increased awareness among staff and student radiographers of the need to produce optimal quality recorded images
    2. Greater care in the production of radiographs because radiographers are aware that the radiographs are being reviewed
    3. Initiation and continuation of in-service education programs for imaging personnel covering problems and concerns identified through the program
    A. 1 only
    B. 2 only
    C. 3 only
    D. 1, 2, and 3

9. Which of the following x-ray beam limitation devices is *most* versatile?
    A. Aperture diaphragm
    B. Radiographic cone
    C. Extension cylinder
    D. Light-localizing variable-aperture rectangular collimator

10. When an individual of childbearing age undergoes a radiologic procedure, gonadal shielding should be used to protect the reproductive organs from exposure to the useful beam
    1. When the reproductive organs are in or within 5 cm of a properly collimated x-ray beam
    2. Unless shielding will compromise the diagnostic value of the examination
    3. When the radiographer chooses to substitute gonadal shielding for adequate collimation of the x-ray beam
    A. 1 and 2 only
    B. 1 and 3 only
    C. 2 and 3 only
    D. 1, 2, and 3

11. Which of the following are *most often* used to assess skin doses?
    A. Compensating filters
    B. Filtration equivalent to 4 mm aluminum in the path of the x-ray beam
    C. Radiographic grids
    D. Thermoluminescent dosimeters

12. Fluoroscopic equipment equipped with HLC may permit a ESE rate *as high as* which of the following?
    A. 5 R/min ($5 \times 2.58 \times 10^{-4}$ C/kg/min)
    B. 10 R/min ($10 \times 2.58 \times 10^{-4}$ C/kg/min)
    C. 20 R/min ($20 \times 2.58 \times 10^{-4}$ C/kg/min)
    D. 50 R/min ($50 \times 2.58 \times 10^{-4}$ C/kg/min)

13. To protect the patient's skin from exposure to electrons produced by photon interaction with the collimator, the skin surface should be at least _____ *below* the collimator.
    A. 6 cm
    B. 12 cm
    C. 15 cm
    D. 20 cm

14. If, in the course of a specific radiographic procedure, 75% of the active bone marrow were in the useful beam and received an average absorbed dose of 0.4 mGy (40 mrads), the mean marrow dose would be which of the following?
    A. 0.3 mGy (30 mrads)
    B. 0.6 mGy (60 mrads)
    C. 0.9 mGy (90 mrads)
    D. 1 mGy (100 rads)

15. Which of the following may reduce patient exposure to off-focus radiation?
    A. Placing the second pair of shutters in the collimator below the level of the light source and mirror
    B. Placing the first pair of shutters in the collimator as close as possible to the x-ray tube window
    C. Transmitting an electric signal through the collimator's first and second pair of shutters
    D. Off-focus radiation in a collimator cannot be reduced

16. Which of the following is an effective technique for reducing patient dose when a digital fluoroscopic system is used?
    A. Converting to nonimage intensification fluoroscopy
    B. Increasing mAs significantly
    C. Using scotopic (rod) vision instead of photopic (cone) vision
    D. Using the last-image-hold feature

17. Compared with patients who undergo cinefluorographic procedures that use lower frame rates, patients who undergo more rapid dynamic function studies (e.g., heart catheterization) receive
    A. Higher radiation doses
    B. Slightly lower radiation doses
    C. Significantly lower radiation doses
    D. Identical radiation doses

18. HLCF is an operating mode for state-of-the-art fluoroscopic equipment in which exposure rates are
    A. Slightly higher than those normally allowed in routine fluoroscopic procedures
    B. Substantially higher than those normally allowed in routine fluoroscopic procedures
    C. Slightly lower than those normally used in routine fluoroscopic procedures
    D. Substantially lower than those normally used in routine fluoroscopic procedures

19. Monitoring and documentation of procedural fluoroscopic time is essential to good practice. The responsibility for monitoring and documentation generally belongs to
    A. The nurse assisting the physician with the procedure
    B. The physician performing the fluoroscopic procedure
    C. The radiographer assisting with the procedure
    D. Radiology department secretarial personnel

20. For all female patients of childbearing age, a gonadal shield should be used when the uterus and ovaries are within the field of view as long as the shield would not impair interpretation of the image. A shield is also recommended if the ovaries and uterus are
   A. More than 5 cm from any edge of the field
   B. Less than 5 cm from any edge of the field
   C. More than 10 cm from any edge of the field
   D. Between 5 and 10 cm from any edge of the field

21. Direct patient shielding is not typically used in
   A. CR
   B. CT
   C. Diagnostic fluoroscopy
   D. Diagnostic radiography

22. Resolution of a digital image is sharper when pixels are
   A. Larger
   B. Smaller
   C. Variable in size
   D. Variable in thickness

23. CT scanning is considered a relatively high radiation exposure diagnostic procedure because of increasing use of
   A. Contrast media
   B. Conventional CT scanners with higher pitch
   C. Multislice spiral (helical) CT scanners using small slice thickness
   D. CT scanners with tighter collimation

24. Compared with the resolution of an optimal quality image produced on radiographic film, the resolution of a digital image is
   A. Actually somewhat less
   B. Comparable to the quality of the imaged produced on radiographic film
   C. Actually somewhat greater
   D. Significantly greater

25. Which of the following radiographic procedures are considered unnecessary?
   1. Chest x-ray as part of a preemployment physical
   2. Chest x-ray examination for mass screening for tuberculosis
   3. Whole-body multislice spiral CT screening
   A. 1 and 2 only
   B. 1 and 3 only
   C. 2 and 3 only
   D. 1, 2, and 3

Exercise 4—True or False

Circle *T* if the statement listed below is true; circle *F* if the statement is false.

1. T F Patient exposure can be substantially reduced by using proper body and/or part immobilization.

2. T F Patients do not need to be given the opportunity to ask questions about their examination when they are having a routine x-ray procedure.

3. T F Radiographic cones, extension cylinders, and aperture diaphragms are x-ray beam filtration devices.

4. T F When PBL is activated, the collimators are automatically adjusted so that the radiation field matches the size of the image receptor.

5. T F Inherent filtration in an x-ray tube used for routine radiography amounts to approximately 2.5-mm aluminum equivalent.

6. T F Because HVL is a measure of beam quality or the effective energy of the x-ray beam, a certain minimal HVL is required at a given peak kilovoltage.

7. T F The lens of the eye, the breasts, and the reproductive organs need not be selectively shielded from the useful beam.

8. T F Primary beam exposure for male patients may be reduced by only 25% when the gonads are covered with a contact shield containing 1 mm of lead.

9. T F To protect the ovaries of a female patient, the shield should be placed approximately 1 inch (2.5 cm) medial to each palpable anterior superior iliac spine.

10. T F Patients with the potential to reproduce should be shielded during x-ray procedures whenever the diagnostic value of the examination is not compromised.

11. T F Use of a lower peak kilovoltage (kVp) and a higher milliamperage and exposure time in seconds (mAs) reduces the patient dose.

12. T F Rare earth screens place less thermal stress on the x-ray tube, increasing its life span.

13. T F When rare earth screens are used, radiation shielding requirements for the x-ray room are increased because a general increase in x-radiation in the environment occurs.

14. T F The patient dose decreases as the grid ratio increases.

15. T F When a radiographic procedure is performed with a CR system, it is acceptable practice to overexpose a patient initially because the image obtained can be technically adjusted to acceptable quality, avoiding the possibility of repeat exposure for the patient.

16. T F Shielding of particularly sensitive breast tissue during a scoliosis examination may be accomplished using a clear lead shadow shield. The radiation dose to the breast of a young patient may be further reduced by performing the scoliosis examination with the x-ray beam entering the anterior surface of the patient's body instead of the posterior surface.

17. T F Poorly processed radiographs offer inadequate diagnostic information, leading to repeat examinations and unnecessary patient exposure.

18. T F Correct matching of screen-film systems is essential; incorrectly matched or incompatible components can result in an increased patient dose.

19. T F Rare earth intensifying screens, which are made of rare earth phosphors (i.e., gadolinium, lanthanum, or yttrium), absorb approximately five times more x-ray energy than the previously used calcium tungstate screens; therefore they emit considerably more light, resulting in a significant reduction in the radiographic exposure required to obtain an image of acceptable quality.

20. T F The use of steel fiber as a front material in a cassette that holds radiographic film and intensifying screens is a recent technologic advancement.

21. T F Compared with conventional screen-film systems, the photostimulable phosphor in the CR imaging plate is much more sensitive to scatter radiation before and after it is sensitized through exposure to a radiographic beam. Because of this increase in sensitivity to scatter radiation, a radiographic grid may be used more frequently during CR imaging.

22. T F Technical exposure factors for fluoroscopic procedures for children require an increase in peak kilovoltage by as much as 25%.

23. T F A primary protective barrier of 2-mm aluminum equivalent is required for an image intensifier unit.

24. T F The use of C-arm fluoroscopy in procedures such as surgical pinning of a fractured hip carries the potential for a relatively large patient radiation dose. C-arm fluoroscope operators, if standing close to the patient, may also be subject to significantly increased occupational exposure with such cases.

25. T F Dose reduction techniques are especially important in cine procedures, which can produce the highest patient doses of all diagnostic procedures. This high dose is caused by a relatively high inherent dose rate and the length of the procedure, particularly in cardiologic (involving cardiac imaging procedures such as heart catheterization) and neuroradiologic studies. Therefore a percentage decrease in the cine dose yields a greater actual dose reduction than the same percentage decrease in non-cine procedures.

Exercise 5—Fill in the Blank

Fill in the blanks with the word or words that best complete the statements below.

1. Radiographers must limit the exposure of the patient to ionizing radiation by using appropriate radiation _____ techniques and _____ devices that _____ radiation exposure.

2. Patient exposure can be substantially reduced by using appropriate beam _____ _____ devices.

3. The radiographer's words and actions must demonstrate understanding and _____ for human dignity and individuality.

4. Repeat radiographic exposures sometimes can be attributed to _____ communication between the radiographer and the patient.

5. Filtration _____ the overall intensity of the radiation.

6. Because of their anatomic location, the _____ reproductive organs receive about three times more exposure during a given radiographic procedure involving the pelvic region than do the _____ reproductive organs.

7. Specific area shielding for selective body areas other than the gonads significantly _____ radiation exposure to those areas and should be used whenever possible.

8. When a male patient is in the supine position, the _____ _____ can be used to guide shield placement over the testes.

9. The _____ filter may be used to provide uniform density when the foot is radiographed in the dorsoplantar projection.

10. With digital radiography, the latent image formed by x-ray photons on a radiation datector is actually a(n) _____ latent image.*

11. Collimating to the anatomic area of interest has the _____ effect in cine as in ordinary fluoroscopy.

12. To limit the effects of inverse fall-off of radiation intensity with _____ during a mobile radiographic examination, a SSD of at least 12 inches (30 cm) must be used.

13. _____ technique charts should be available for each x-ray unit to help provide a uniform selection of technical exposure factors. _____ kVp and _____ mAs should be chosen whenever possible to reduce the amount of radiation received by the patient yet maintain acceptable radiographic contrast.

14. Adequate collimation of the radiographic beam to include only the area of _____ _____ is essential.

15. The estimated GSD for the U.S. population is about _____ mSv (_____ mrem).

16. Primary beam exposure for male patients may be reduced as much as _____% to _____% when the gonads are covered with a contact shield containing 1 mm of lead.

17. Suspended from above the radiographic beam defining system, shadow shields hang over the area of clinical interest to cast a _____ in the primary beam over the patient's reproductive organs.

18. Selection of appropriate technical exposure factors for each x-ray examination is essential to ensure a diagnostic image with _____ patient dose.

19. In digital radiography the numeric value in each miniature square box that comprises the image matrix can be converted into a visual brightness, or _____ level, that can be seen on a video display monitor.

20. Digital radiographic images can be accessed at several _____ at the same time, which makes image viewing convenient for physicians providing patient care.

21. With CR, overexposing patients to possibly avoid repeat radiographic exposures is _____ _____ and _____.

22. Because an image intensification system greatly increases brightness, image intensification fluoroscopy requires less milliamperage than does old-fashioned conventional fluoroscopy. The consequent decrease in the exposure rate can result in a sizable _____ _____ for the patient.

23. The fluoroscopic exposure control switch (e.g., foot pedal) must be of the _____ type (i.e., only continuous pressure applied by the operator can keep the switch activated and the fluoroscopic tube emitting x-radiation).

24. When the SSD is small (e.g., for mobile radiographic examinations), patient _____ exposure is significantly greater than _____ _____ exposure. By increasing the SSD, the radiographer maintains a more uniform distribution of exposure throughout the patient.

25. Whenever a female patient of childbearing age is to undergo an x-ray examination, it is essential that the radiographer carefully question the patient about the possibility of _____. Part of this questioning involves asking the patient for the date of her last _____ _____.

*Bushong SC: *Radiologic science for technologists: Physics, biology, and protection*, ed 8, p. 589, St. Louis, 2004, Mosby.

109

Exercise 6—Labeling

Label the following illustrations and table.

A. X-ray tube, collimator, and image receptor.

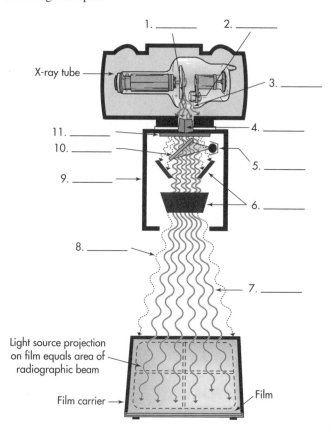

B. Image intensification fluoroscopic unit.

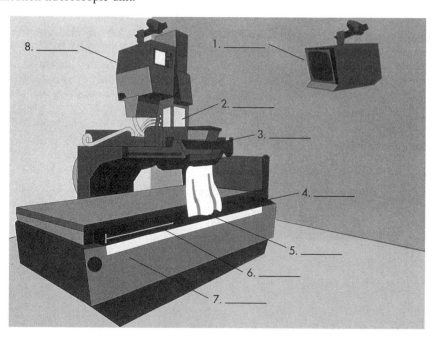

From *Mosby's radiographic instructional series: radiobiology and radiation protection*, St Louis, 1999, Mosby.

Chapter **8** **Protection of the Patient During Diagnostic X-Ray Procedures**

C. HVL required by the Radiation Control for Health and Safety Act of 1968 and detailed by the Bureau of Radiological Health* in 1980

Peak Kilovoltage	Minimum Required HVL in Millimeters of Aluminum
30	1._____
40	2._____
50	3._____
60	4._____
70	5._____
80	6._____
90	7._____
100	8._____
110	9._____
120	10._____

*The Bureau of Radiological Health changed its name to the Center for Devices and Radiological Health in 1982.

Exercise 7—Short Answer

Answer the following questions by providing a short answer.

1. How can radiographers limit exposure of the patient to ionizing radiation during a radiographic procedure?

_____

_____

2. Why is it impossible to eliminate all off-focus, or stem, radiation coming from the primary beam and exiting at various angles from the x-ray tube window?

_____

_____

3. List four basic types of gonadal shielding devices that can be used during a radiologic procedure.

_____

_____

4. What is the direct consequence of poorly processed radiographs?

_____

_____

111

5. What is protective shielding?

_____

_____

6. How is an air gap technique performed? How does use of this technique for certain examinations help reduce scattered x-rays? How does the patient dose received from an air gap technique compare with the dose received from use of a midratio grid?

_____

_____

7. What does inherent filtration include?

_____

_____

8. List three reasons for high radiation exposure during an interventional procedure performed by a physician who is not a radiologist.

_____

_____

9. List four ways to specify the amount of radiation a patient receives from a diagnostic imaging procedure.

_____

_____

10. Why is direct patient shielding not typically used in CT?

_____

_____

11. How does filtration reduce the overall intensity of radiation in a radiographic beam?

_____

_____

12. With regard to the diagnostic x-ray tube, where is added filtration located?

_____

_____

13. List seven factors that must be considered in the selection of technical exposure.

_____

_____

14. List three benefits of a repeat analysis program.

_____

_____

15. List six x-ray procedures that are now considered nonessential.

_____

_____

16. List seven categories that may be established for discarded radiographs.

_____

_____

17. List eleven procedures involving extended fluoroscopic time.

_____

_____

18. Why is a cumulative timing device needed on fluoroscopic equipment?

_____

_____

19. For dose reduction purposes, why is it best to position the C-arm of a C-arm fluoroscopic unit so that the x-ray tube is under the patient whenever possible?

_____

_____

20. How are thermoluminescent dosimeters (TLDs) used to measure skin dose directly?

_____

_____

Exercise 8—Essay

On a separate sheet of paper, answer the following questions in essay form.

1. Describe the procedures that should be followed if a pregnant patient is irradiated inadvertently.

2. Describe strategies that can be used to manage the radiation dose to patients and x-ray equipment operators and staff during interventional fluoroscopy.

3. Discuss the use of fluoroscopic equipment by physicians who are not radiologists from a radiation safety point of view.

4. Discuss the value of effective communication between the radiographer and patient as it relates to radiation safety during a diagnostic x-ray examination.

5. Discuss the potential for radiogenic skin injuries during fluoroscopically guided therapeutic interventional procedures.

Chapter **8** **Protection of the Patient During Diagnostic X-Ray Procedures**

The student should take this test after reading Chapter 8, finishing all accompanying textbook and workbook exercises, and completing any additional activities required by the course instructor. The student should complete the post test with a score of 90% or higher before advancing to the next chapter. (Each of the following 20 questions or blanks is worth 5 points.) Score = _____ %

1. Current federal standards limit ESE rates of general purpose intensified fluoroscopic units to a maximum of _____ R/min.

2. What is the current position of the American College of Radiology (ACR) regarding abdominal radiologic examinations that have been requested by a physician after full consideration of the clinical status of a patient, including the possibility of pregnancy?

   _____

   _____

3. Whenever a repeat radiograph must be taken as a consequence of human or mechanical error, the skin and gonads of the patient receive a _____ _____ of x-radiation.

4. What is the most versatile x-ray beam limitation device currently in use?

   _____

   _____

5. Define the term *genetically significant dose.*

   _____

   _____

6. How does the use of a radiographic grid affect the patient dose?

   _____

   _____

7. When verbal messages and unconscious actions, or body language (i.e., nonverbal messages), are understood as intended, communication between the radiographer and patient is _____.

8. Which of the following substantially reduces patient exposure?
   1. Use of proper body and/or part immobilization
   2. Use of appropriate beam limitation devices
   3. Use of gonadal or other specific area shielding
   A. 1 and 2 only
   B. 1 and 3 only
   C. 2 and 3 only
   D. 1, 2, and 3

9. Filtration that includes the glass envelope encasing the x-ray tube, the insulating oil surrounding the tube, and the glass window in the tube housing is called
   A. Added filtration
   B. Inherent filtration
   C. Total filtration
   D. HVL

114

10. Gonadal shielding should be a secondary protective measure, not a substitute for an adequately _____ beam.

11. Compared with slower rare earth film-screen image receptors, faster rare earth film-screen image receptor systems can demonstrate an effect referred to as _____ _____.

12. HLCF is used for what purpose?

_____

13. Correctly placed, appropriate gonadal shielding can greatly reduce the exposure received by both genders (_____% for females, 90% to 95% for males).

14. What fluoroscopic practice should a radiologist use to reduce the overall length of the exposure for a given procedure?

_____

_____

15. To protect the patient's skin from exposure to electrons produced by photon interaction with the collimator, the skin surface should be at least _____ cm below the collimator.
    A. 3
    B. 5
    C. 10
    D. 15

16. To what must the alignment and the length and width dimensions of the radiographic and light beams correspond?

_____

_____

17. Because of their anatomic location, the female reproductive organs receive about _____ times more exposure during a radiographic procedure involving the pelvic region than do the male reproductive organs.

18. What external anatomic landmark can a radiographer use for placement of a testicular shield on a male patient in the supine position?

_____

_____

19. Placing the first pair of shutters in the collimator as close as possible to the x-ray tube window may
    A. Eliminate the need for a second pair of shutters
    B. Eliminate the need for added filtration
    C. Reduce patient exposure from the primary beam
    D. Reduce patient exposure from off-focus, or stem, radiation

20. Dose reduction in mammography can be achieved by limiting the number of _____ taken.

9 Protection of Imaging Personnel During Diagnostic X-Ray Procedures

Radiographers may be exposed to secondary radiation (scatter and leakage) while fulfilling professional responsibilities associated with diagnostic imaging. This increases their occupational exposure. Chapter 9 presents an overview of methods to reduce this exposure. Diagnostic x-ray suite protection design is also covered, with emphasis on new approaches to shielding in accordance with National Council of Radiation Protection and Measurements (NCRP) Report No. 147.

CHAPTER HIGHLIGHTS

- An annual occupational effective dose (EfD) of 50 mSv (5 rem) for whole-body exposure during routine operations and an annual EfD of 1 mSv (0.1 rem) for members of the general population has been established.
- A cumulative effective dose (CumEfD) limits a radiation worker's whole-body lifetime EfD to the person's age multiplied by 10 mSv (years × 1 rem).
- Radiation workers can receive a larger equivalent dose (EqD) than the general public without altering the genetically significant dose (GSD).
- Occupational exposure must be kept as low as reasonably achievable (ALARA).
- The following methods of reducing scatter radiation also reduce the occupational hazard for the radiographer:
  - Use of beam-limitation devices, higher kVp and lower mAs techniques, appropriate beam filtration, and adequate protective shielding
  - Correct use of protective apparel (i.e., lead aprons, gloves, thyroid shields)
  - Reduction of repeat examinations
- The basic principles of time, distance, and shielding can be used to minimize occupational radiation exposure.
- Pregnant radiographers can wear an additional monitoring device at waist level to ensure that the monthly EqD does not exceed 0.5 mSv (0.05 rem).
- Primary and secondary protective barriers must be designed to ensure that the annual EfD limits are not exceeded.
- Lead-lined, metal, diagnostic-type protective tube housing must be used to protect the radiographer and patient from leakage radiation.

- The following measures should be taken to protect the radiographer during routine fluoroscopy:
  - In addition to wearing appropriate protective apparel, the radiographer should stand as far from the patient as is practical and move closer to the patient only when assistance is required.
  - A spot film device protective curtain and a Bucky slot shielding device must be used.
  - The x-ray beam must be adequately collimated, and high-speed image receptor systems and a cumulative timing device should also be used.
- Radiographers should take the following measures to protect themselves during mobile radiographic examinations:
  - Wear protective garments
  - Stand at least 6 feet (1.8 m) from the patient, x-ray tube, and useful beam
  - Stand at a right angle to the x-ray beam–scattering object (the patient) line
- Limited exposure time and dose reduction features are required to protect the radiographer during high-level-control fluoroscopy.
- Distance is the most effective means of protection from ionizing radiation.
- If the peak energy of the x-ray beam is 100 kVp, a lead apron of at least 0.25-mm lead-equivalent thickness should be worn if the radiographer cannot remain behind a protective barrier. A lead apron of 0.5 or 1-mm lead equivalent affords much greater protection.
- Lead gloves, a thyroid shield, and protective glasses sometimes are required.
- Radiographers should never stand in the primary beam to hold a patient during a radiographic exposure.
- When diagnostic x-ray suites are designed, the EqD to radiation workers, nonoccupationally exposed personnel, and the general public must be taken into consideration.
  - Facilities must be equipped with radiation-absorbent barriers.
  - The occupancy factor, workload, and use factor must be considered in the determination of thickness requirements for a protective barrier. Whether an area beyond a structure is designated as a controlled or an uncontrolled area is a significant factor in determining the amount of radiation shielding to be added to the structure.

116

Exercise 1—Crossword Puzzle

Use the clues to complete the crossword puzzle.

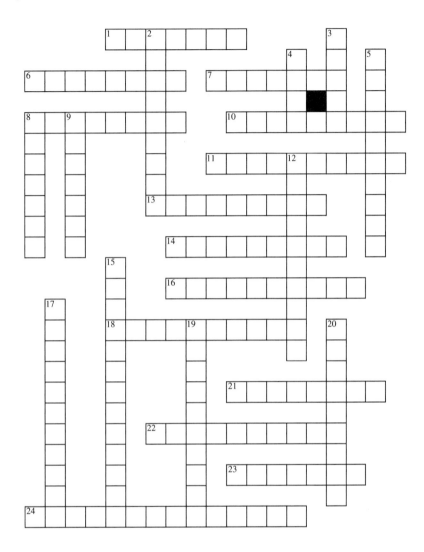

Down

2. The effect on the radiation dose as the length of exposure time shortens.
3. Accessory protective device made of lead-impregnated vinyl.
4. Scheduling radiographers to assigned clinical areas in a rotational pattern uses this cardinal principle as a means of radiation protection.
5. Primarily benefits the patient.
8. Source of scattered radiation during a diagnostic x-ray procedure.
9. Type of secondary radiation.
12. The designation for an area adjacent to a wall of an x-ray room that is used only by occupationally exposed personnel.
15. How primary protective barriers are located in relation to the un-deflected line of travel of the x-ray beam.
17. Term used when a pregnant technologist first informs her supervisor that she is pregnant.
19. Dose that is the product of the average absorbed does in a tissue or organ in the human body and its associated radiation weighting factor, chosen for the type and energy of the radiation in question for radiation workers.
20. Type of protective barrier that a control-booth barrier is considered to be.

Chapter **9** **Protection of Imaging Personnel During Diagnostic X-Ray Procedures**

Across

1. Type of personal exposure that a radiographer's effective dose does not include.
6. The most effective means of protection from ionizing radiation.
7. A thickness that radiographers are not required to determine.
8. Established by health care facilities to protect pregnant personnel from radiation.
10. Type of protective apparel that should be available for pregnant radiologists and radiographers.
11. Type of radiation-absorbent barriers such as walls and doors.
13. When it is not possible to use the cardinal principles of time or distance to minimize occupational exposure, this may be used to provide protection from radiation.

14. Type of radiation that poses the greatest occupational hazard in diagnostic radiology.
16. What a pregnant radiologic technologist must receive, after she informs a supervisor she is pregnant.
18. Type of eyeglasses that can be worn to reduce scattered radiation to the lens of the eyes.
21. Quantity that best describes the weekly radiation usage of a diagnostic x-ray unit.
22. Type of protective apron that can be work for protection during pregnancy.
23. Radiation that emerges directly from the x-ray tube collimator.
24. Type of procedures that use high-level-control fluoroscopy.

Exercise 2—Matching

Match the following terms with their definitions or associated phrases.

1. _____ 50 mSv (5 rem)

2. _____ control booth barrier
3. _____ 0.5 mSv (0.05 rem)
4. _____ ALARA concept

5. _____ diagnostic-type protective tube housing
6. _____ secondary radiation

7. _____ workload (W)
8. _____ spot film device protective curtain

9. _____ CumEfD limit

10. _____ occupancy factor (T)

11. _____ Bucky slot shielding device

12. _____ GSD

13. _____ inverse square law (ISL)

14. _____ use factor (U)

15. _____ scatter radiation

16. _____ protective eyeglasses

17. _____ secondary protective barrier

18. _____ high-level-control

A. The intensity of radiation is inversely proportional to the square of the distance from the source.
B. Protects against leakage and scatter radiation
C. Annual occupational EfD limit
D. Possibility of developing a radiogenic cancer or the induction of a genetic defect as a consequence of radiation exposure
E. Prevents direct, or unscattered, radiation from reaching personnel on the other side
F. Monthly allowance EqD to the embryo-fetus from occupational exposure of a pregnant technologist
G. Beam direction factor
H. Annual EqD limit to localized areas of the skin and hands
I. Specified in units of milliampere-seconds (mAs) per week or milliampere-minutes (mA-min) per week
J. Automatically covers the Bucky slot opening in the side of the x-ray table during a standard fluoroscopic examination when the Bucky tray is positioned at the foot end of the table
K. Required to protect both the radiographer and the patient from off-focus, or leakage, radiation by restricting the emission of x-rays to the area of the useful beam
L. Used to modify the shielding requirement for a particular barrier by taking into account the fraction of the workweek that the space beyond the barrier is occupied
M. Permits the radiologist and assisting radiographer to remain outside the fluoroscopic room at a control console behind a protective barrier until needed
N. Mode of operation in which the exposure rate may significantly exceed the rate used in routine fluoroscopy
O. Should be positioned between the fluoroscopist and the patient to intercept scattered radiation above the tabletop during a fluoroscopic examination
P. A permanent protective barrier for the radiographer that is located in an x-ray room housing stationary (fixed) radiographic equipment
Q. A radiation worker's whole-body lifetime EfD must be limited to the person's age in years multiplied by 10 mSv (years × 1 rem).
R. All the radiation that arises from interactions of an x-ray beam with the atoms of an object in the path of the beam

19. _____ protective apparel

S. Principle that holds that occupational exposure of the radiographer and other occupationally exposed persons should be kept as low as reasonably achievable

20. _____ remote control fluoroscopic system

T. The EqD to the reproductive organs that, if received by every human being, would be expected to cause an identical gross genetic injury to the total population as does the sum of the actual doses received by exposed individual population members

21. _____ primary protective barrier

U. The radiation that results from the interaction between primary radiation and the atoms of the irradiated object and the off-focus or leakage radiation that penetrates the x-ray tube protective housing; this radiation consists of scattered radiation and leakage radiation

22. _____ C-arm fluoroscope

V. Glasses with optically clear lenses that contain a minimal lead equivalent protection of 0.35 mm

23. _____ 500 mSv (50 rem)

W. X-rays emitted through the x-ray tube window or port

24. _____ occupational risk

X. Special garments (e.g., aprons, gloves, and thyroid shields) that conventionally are made of lead-impregnated vinyl and are worn during fluoroscopic and certain radiographic procedures

25. _____ useful (primary) beam

Y. A portable device for producing real-time (motion) images of a patient; this device holds an x-ray tube at one end and a image intensifier at the other end

Exercise 3—Multiple Choice

Select the answer that best completes the following questions or statements.

1. Because the workforce in radiation-related jobs is small compared with the population as a whole, the amount of radiation received by this workforce can be larger than the amount received by the general public without altering the
   A. GSD
   B. Lethal dose (LD) 50/30
   C. Mean marrow dose (MMD)
   D. Tumor induction risk ratio (TIRR)

2. Which of the following is a tenet of the ALARA concept?
   A. The radiographer's occupational exposure should not exceed the annual EfD limit allowed for individual members of the general population.
   B. The radiographer's occupational exposure should be as high as necessary to allow for holding of patients during diagnostic x-ray procedures.
   C. The radiographer's occupational exposure for the whole body should limit that individual's lifetime EfD to the person's age multiplied by 50 mSv (years × 5 rem).
   D. The radiographer's exposure should be kept as low as reasonably achievable.

3. A facility that employs a pregnant diagnostic imaging staff member should provide that individual with an additional monitor to be worn at waist level during *all* radiation procedures. The purpose of this additional monitor is to ensure that the monthly EqD to the embryo-fetus does not exceed
   A. 50 mSv (5 rem)
   B. 10 mSv (1 rem)
   C. 5 mSv (0.5 rem)
   D. 0.5 mSv (0.05 rem)

4. Which of the following are radiation sources that can be generated in a diagnostic x-ray room?
   1. Primary radiation
   2. Scatter radiation
   3. Leakage radiation
   A. 1 only
   B. 2 only
   C. 3 only
   D. 1, 2, and 3

5. During C-arm fluoroscopy, the exposure rate caused by scatter near the entrance surface of the patient (the x-ray tube side) _____ the exposure rate caused by scatter near the exit surface of the patient (the image intensifier side).
   A. Equals
   B. Exceeds
   C. Is slightly less than
   D. Is considerably less than

6. For high-level-control interventional procedures, the radiographer should verify that which of the following dose reduction features are available and in good working order?
   1. High-quality, low-dose fluoroscopy mode and pulsed radiation mode
   2. Collimation and filtration
   3. Roadmapping, time-interval differences, and last-image-hold features
   A. 1 only
   B. 2 only
   C. 3 only
   D. 1, 2, and 3

7. In diagnostic radiology, which of the following radiation sources poses the *greatest* occupational hazard for the radiographer?
   A. Image-formation radiation
   B. Leakage radiation
   C. Primary radiation
   D. Scattered radiation

8. Which of the following methods and devices reduce(s) the radiographer's exposure during a fluoroscopic examination?
   1. Adequate x-ray beam collimation
   2. Control of technical exposure factors
   3. Gonadal shielding of the patient
   A. 1 only
   B. 2 only
   C. 3 only
   D. 1, 2, and 3

9. If the peak energy of the diagnostic x-ray beam is 130 kVp, the primary protective barrier generally should consist of at least _____ and extend _____ upward from the floor of the x-ray room when the tube is 5 to 7 feet from the wall in question.
   A. 1/16 inch lead, 7 feet
   B. 1/16 inch lead, 10 feet
   C. 1/32 inch lead, 7 feet
   D. 1/32 inch lead, 10 feet

10. Which of the following radiation sources is the control booth barrier *not* intended to intercept in a diagnostic x-ray room?
    1. Leakage radiation
    2. Primary radiation
    3. Scattered radiation
    A. 1 only
    B. 2 only
    C. 3 only
    D. 1 and 3

11. Protective shielding for an uncontrolled area (e.g., a hall or corridor frequented by the general public) must ensure that the maximal EqD for that area is *no greater than* _____ per week.
    A. 1000 microsievert (100 mrem)
    B. 100 microsievert (10 mrem)
    C. 20 microsievert (2 mrem)
    D. 10 microsievert (1 mrem)

12. Which of the following statements is *true?*
    A. If wearing a protective apron, a radiographer may stand in the useful beam to restrain a patient during a difficult radiologic procedure.
    B. If wearing protective aprons, nurses, orderlies, relatives, or friends may stand in the useful beam to restrain a patient during a difficult radiologic procedure.
    C. If wearing protective aprons, pregnant radiographers or other nonoccupationally exposed pregnant females may stand in the useful beam to restrain a patient during a difficult radiologic procedure.
    D. Radiographers and nonoccupationally exposed individuals should never stand in the useful beam to restrain a patient during a radiographic procedure.

13. Of the devices listed below, which eliminates low-energy photons in the collimator to *reduce* scattered radiation potential?
    1. Collimator light source
    2. Electronic sensors
    3. Aluminum filtration
    A. 1 only
    B. 2 only
    C. 3 only
    D. 1, 2, and 3

14. Which of the following is the *most effective* means of protection from ionizing radiation normally available to the radiographer?
    A. Reducing the amount of time spent near a source of radiation
    B. Placing as much distance as possible between oneself and the source of radiation
    C. Remaining behind a mobile protective shield during an exposure
    D. Using protective shielding garments

15. The lead glass window of the control booth barrier in a stationary (fixed) radiographic installation typically consists of which of the following?
    A. 0.25 mm lead equivalent
    B. 0.5 mm lead equivalent
    C. 1 mm lead equivalent
    D. 1.5 mm lead equivalent

16. The beam direction factor is also known as the
    A. Occupancy factor
    B. ISL
    C. Workload
    D. Use factor

17. If the intensity of the x-ray is inversely proportional to the square of the distance from the source, how does the intensity of the x-ray beam change when the distance from the source of radiation and a measurement point is quadrupled?
    A. It increases by a factor of 4 at the new distance.
    B. It increases by a factor of 16 at the new distance.
    C. It decreases by a factor of 16 at the new distance.
    D. It decreases by a factor of 4 at the new distance.

120

18. Leakage radiation and scatter radiation are forms of
    A. Cosmic radiation
    B. Natural background radiation
    C. Nonionizing radiation
    D. Secondary radiation

19. Diagnostic x-ray installations must be equipped with
    A. Barriers made of aluminum
    B. Barriers made of Sheetrock
    C. Radiation-absorbent barriers
    D. Radiation-nonabsorbent barriers

20. Which of the following principles can be used to minimize occupational radiation exposure?
    1. Time
    2. Distance
    3. Shielding
    A. 1 and 2 only
    B. 1 and 3 only
    C. 2 and 3 only
    D. 1, 2, and 3

21. Pregnant radiographers can wear an additional monitoring device at waist level to ensure that the monthly EqD does not exceed
    A. 0.1 mSv (0.01 rem)
    B. 0.2 mSv (0.02 rem)
    C. 0.3 mSv (0.03 rem)
    D. 0.5 mSv (0.05 rem)

22. During fluoroscopy, which of the following will provide radiation protection for the radiographer and the radiologist?
    1. Adequate collimation of the x-ray beam
    2. Use of high-speed image receptor systems
    3. Use of cumulative timing device
    A. 1 and 2 only
    B. 1 and 3 only
    C. 2 and 3 only
    D. 1, 2, and 3

23. Floors of radiation rooms except dental installations, doors, walls, and ceilings of radiation rooms exposed routinely to the primary beam are given a use factor of
    A. 1
    B. 1/2
    C. 1/4
    D. 1/16

24. If a radiographer stands 1 m from an x-ray tube and is subject to an exposure rate of 4 mR/hr, what will the exposure rate be if the same radiographer moves to a position 2 m from the x-ray tube?
    A. 1 mR/hr
    B. 2 mR/hr
    C. 8 mR/hr
    D. 16 mR/hr

25. If a radiographer moves closer to a source of radiation, the radiation exposure to the radiographer
    A. Decreases slightly
    B. Decreases significantly
    C. Increases slightly
    D. Increases significantly

Exercise 4—True or False

Circle *T* if the statement listed below is true; circle *F* if the statement is false.

1. T F General fluoroscopy increases the radiographer's risk of exposure to ionizing radiation.

2. T F A radiographer's annual occupational EfD includes personal medical and natural background radiation exposure.

3. T F The ALARA concept takes economic and social factors into consideration.

4. T F Protective lead aprons and shielded barriers function as gonadal shields for diagnostic imaging personnel.

5. T F The intensity of radiation is directly proportional to the square of the distance from the source.

6. T F Clear lead-plastic overhead protective barriers used as an overhead x-ray barrier typically offer 2-mm lead equivalent protection.

7. T F If the peak energy of an x-ray beam is 100 kVp, a protective lead (Pb) apron must be equivalent to at least 0.5-mm thickness of lead.

8. T F If the radiographer's immediate presence assisting a radiologist during a fluoroscopic examination is not required near the x-ray table, this person may stand behind the radiologist who is wearing protective apparel.

9. T F The spot film device protective curtain protects the radiologist and radiographer at the gonadal level.

10. T F For C-arm devices with similar fields of view, the dose rate to personnel within 1 m of the patient is comparable to that of routine fluoroscopy.

11. T F The physical configuration of a C-arm fluoroscopic unit allows for many methods of achieving protection from scattered radiation.

12. T F From the perspective of increased radiation safety, it is best to reverse the C-arm to place the x-ray tube under the table and the image intensifier over the table.

13. T F A radiographer may hold a patient during a radiographic exposure as long as the radiographer stands in the useful beam.

14. T F In a typical x-ray suite, the most common primary radiation barrier is that behind the wall Bucky unit.

15. T F Because scatter and leakage radiation emerge in all directions in the x-ray room, every wall, door, viewing window, and other surface is always struck by some amount of radiation.

16. T F Filtration primarily benefits the radiographer.

17. T F During a diagnostic x-ray procedure, the patient becomes a source of scattered radiation as a consequence of the coherent scattering process.

18. T F At a 90-degree angle to the primary x-ray beam, at a distance of 1 m, the scattered x-ray intensity generally is approximately $1/1000$ of the intensity of the primary x-ray beam.

19. T F Methods and techniques that reduce patient exposure also reduce exposure for the radiographer.

20. T F Pregnant diagnostic imaging department staff members must immediately stop performing their respective duties and immediately discontinue employment as a consequence of pregnancy.

21. T F The amount of radiation a worker receives is inversely proportional to the length of time the individual is exposed to ionizing radiation.

22. T F If a declared pregnant radiographer is reassigned to a lower radiation exposure risk area, other unknowing, potentially pregnant radiographers can be subject to increased risk. Therefore the declared pregnant radiographer does not necessarily need to be reassigned to a lower radiation exposure as a direct consequence of a declared pregnancy.

23. T F In accordance with ALARA guidelines, work schedules are designed to evenly distribute radiation exposure risk to all employees.

24. T F In a typical x-ray room, a secondary barrier should overlap the primary barrier by about $1/2$ inch (1.25 cm).

25. T F A radiographer need not wear a protective apron during a fluoroscopic examination.

Exercise 5—Fill in the Blank

Fill in the blanks with the word or words that best complete the statements below.

1. Although the radiographer and other diagnostic imaging personnel are allowed to absorb more radiation than the general public, the _____ dose received must be minimized whenever possible.

2. _____ radiation poses the greatest occupational hazard in diagnostic radiology.

3. The use of correct radiographic film processing techniques leads to a _____ in the number of repeat examinations required, with a resultant _____ in exposure to the radiographer.

4. After receiving radiation safety counseling, a pregnant radiologic technologist must read and sign a form acknowledging that she has received counseling and understands the ways to implement appropriate measures to ensure the _____ of the embryo-fetus.

5. If a declared pregnant radiographer is reassigned to a lower radiation exposure risk area, other unknowing potentially pregnant radiographers can be subject to _____ risk.

6. _____ the length of time spent in a room where x-radiation is produced reduces occupational exposure.

7. The most effective means of protection from ionizing radiation is _____.

8. Structural barriers such as walls and doors in an x-ray room provide radiation _____ _____ for both imaging department personnel and the general public.

9. Accessory protective shielding includes _____, _____, and _____ _____ made of lead-impregnated vinyl.

10. No one should touch the tube _____ or _____ cables while a radiographic exposure is in progress.

11. When high-speed image receptor systems are used, smaller radiographic exposure (less milliamperage) is required, which results in fewer x-ray photons being available to produce _____ _____. Because of this reduction in _____ _____, personnel exposure is decreased.

12. It is imperative that the EqD to the embryo-fetus from occupational exposure of the mother not exceed the NCRP-recommended monthly EqD limit of _____ mSv (_____ rem) or a limit of _____ mSv (_____ rem) during the entire pregnancy.

13. Maternity protective aprons consist of _____ lead equivalent over their entire length and width, and also have an extra _____ lead equivalent protective panel that runs transversely across the width of the apron to provide added safety for the embryo-fetus.

14. Shortening the length of _____ spent in a room where x-radiation is produced, standing at the greatest _____ possible from an energized x-ray beam, and interposing a radiation-absorbent _____ material between the radiation worker and the source of radiation all reduce occupational exposure.

15. When the distance from the x-ray target, a point source of radiation, is doubled, the radiation at the new location spans an area _____ times larger than the original area. However, because the same amount of radiation exists to cover this larger area, the intensity (amount, or quantity, of radiation) at the new distance decreases by a factor of _____.

16. Primary protective barriers are located _____ _____ to the undeflected line of travel of the x-ray beam.

17. If the peak energy of the x-ray beam is 130 kVp, the primary protective barrier in a typical installation consists of _____ lead and extends _____ feet (___ m) upward from the floor of the x-ray room when the x-ray tube is 5 to 7 feet from the wall in question.

18. In a typical diagnostic x-ray installation, the secondary barrier consists of _____ lead.

19. During fluoroscopy and x-ray special procedures, a neck and thyroid shield can guard the thyroid area

of occupationally exposed people. It should be _____ lead equivalent.

20. To ensure protection from _____ radiation emanating from the patient during a fluoroscopic examination, the radiographer should stand as far from the _____ as is practical and should move closer to the patient only when _____ is required.

21. Protective lead gloves of at least _____ lead equivalent should be worn whenever the hands must be placed near the fluoroscopic field.

22. If the radiographer's immediate presence in assisting a radiologist during a fluoroscopic examination is not required near the x-ray table, the radiographer should stand behind the _____, who is also wearing protective apparel, or should stand behind the _____ _____ until his or her services are required.

23. A _____ protective apron is recommended to protect personnel who must move around the x-ray room during a fluoroscopic examination.

24. The radiographer should attempt to stand at _____ _____ (___ degrees) to the x-ray beam scattering object (the patient) line; when the protective factors of distance and shielding have been accounted for, this is the place where the _____ amount of scattered radiation is received.

25. For C-arm fluoroscopes with similar fields of view, the dose rate to personnel within 1 m of the patient is comparable to that of _____ fluoroscopy, approximately several mGy/hr.

Exercise 6—Labeling

Label the following illustrations.

A. Relationship between distance and intensity.

| More distance | = | Less intensity (quantity of radiation) |

| 2 × d | = | 1. _____ |

| 3 × d | = | 2. _____ |

| 4 × d | = | 3. _____ |

B. Protective barriers.

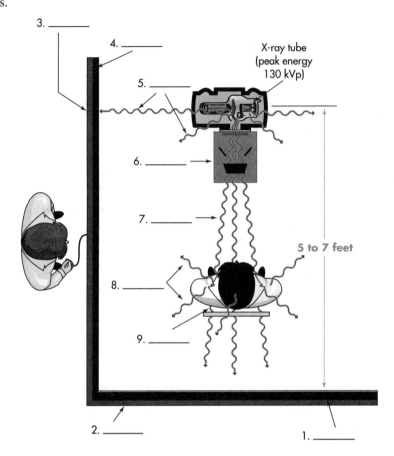

X-ray tube
(peak energy
130 kVp)

5 to 7 feet

C. Standing at right angles to the scattering object.

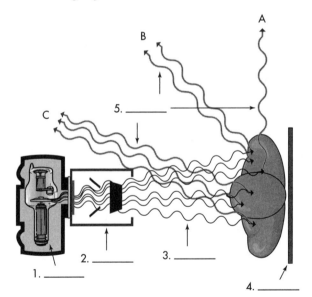

Chapter **9** **Protection of Imaging Personnel During Diagnostic X-Ray Procedures**

Exercise 7—Short Answer

Answer the following questions by providing a short answer.

1. With what occupational groups are monitored diagnostic imaging personnel compared for the purpose of assessing occupational risk?

_____

_____

2. From what types of x-radiation are lead aprons designed to provide protection?

_____

_____

3. How does the use of high-speed imaging receptor systems help reduce occupational exposure of the radiographer?

_____

_____

4. Why should a pregnant radiographer "declare" a pregnancy?

_____

_____

5. List the three basic principles of radiation protection.

_____

_____

6. Who should determine the exact requirements for protective structural shielding for a particular imaging facility?

_____

_____

7. Protective aprons, gloves, and thyroid shields are made of what material?

_____

_____

8. How can scattered radiation to the lens of the eyes of diagnostic imaging personnel be substantially reduced?

_____

_____

9. How does a lead-lined, metal, diagnostic-type protective tube housing protect the radiographer and the patient from off-focus, or leakage, radiation?

_____

_____

Chapter **9** **Protection of Imaging Personnel During Diagnostic X-Ray Procedures**

10. How does the use of a remote control fluoroscopic unit increase the safety of imaging personnel?

_____

_____

11. From the perspective of increased radiation safety, why is it best to place the x-ray tube end of the C-arm under the table and the image intensifier over the table whenever possible?

_____

_____

12. During operating room procedures in which cross-table exposures are obtained with a mobile C-arm fluoroscope, where is the potential for scatter dose lower in relation to the patient?

_____

_____

13. How can the radiologist or other interventional physician reduce radiation exposure during a high-level-control interventional procedure?

_____

_____

14. Why should physicians performing interventional procedures wear extremity monitors? What is the annual EqD limit for localized areas of the skin and hands? What can physicians use to protect their hands during an interventional procedure?

_____

_____

15. List eight radiation-absorbent barrier design considerations.

_____

_____

Exercise 8—Essay

On a separate sheet of paper, answer the following questions in essay form.

1. Discuss the importance of protective structural shielding in an imaging facility.

2. Describe various dose reduction methods and techniques that may be used effectively to protect the radiographer.

3. Describe in detail the various types of protective apparel available for personnel in most health care facilities and give examples of the appropriate use of each item.

4. Describe radiation protection problems that a radiographer might encounter when performing a mobile radiographic examination. Explain how each problem can be safely resolved.

5. Describe radiation protection problems that a radiographer may encounter when operating a mobile C-arm fluoroscope in the operating room. Explain how each problem can be safely resolved.

Exercise 9—Calculation Problems

Solve the following problems.

The ISL expresses the relationship between the distance and the intensity (quantity) of radiation. The law states: The intensity of radiation is inversely proportional to the square of the distance from the source. To be more precise, as the distance between the radiation source and a measurement point increases, the quantity of radiation measured at the more distant position decreases by the square of the ratio of the original distance from the source to that of the new distance from the source.

This decrease in radiation physically occurs because the area, which the same flux of x-rays at the original location now covers at the new location, has increased by the square of the relative distance change. For example, as demonstrated in the illustration that follows, when the distance from the x-ray target, a point source of radiation, is doubled, the radiation at the new location spans an area four times larger than the original area. However, because the same amount of radiation exists to cover this larger area, the intensity at the new distance consequently decreases by a factor of four.

The ISL may be stated as a formula, shown in the following equation. A mathematical example is also provided.

$$\frac{I_1}{I_2} = \frac{(d_2)^2}{(d_1)^2}$$

Where I_1 expresses the exposure (intensity) at the original distance; I_2 expresses the exposure (intensity) at the new distance; d_1 expresses the original distance from the source of radiation; and d_2 expresses the new distance from the source of radiation.

Example: If a radiographer stands 2 m from an x-ray tube and is subject to an exposure rate of 6 mR/hr, what will the exposure rate be if the same radiographer moves to a position 4 m from the x-ray tube?

Answer:

$$\frac{I_1}{I_2} = \frac{(d_2)^2}{(d_1)^2}$$

$$\frac{6}{I_2} = \frac{(4)^2}{(2)^2}$$

$$\frac{6}{I_2} = \frac{16}{4} \text{ (cross multiply)}$$

$$16\,I_2 = 24$$

$$I_2 = 1.5\,\text{mR/hr}$$

1. If a radiographer stands 3 m from an x-ray tube and is subject to an exposure rate of 9 mR/hr, what will the exposure rate be if the same radiographer moves to a position 6 m from the x-ray tube?

2. If a radiographer stands 2 feet from an x-ray tube and is subject to an exposure rate of 5 mR/hr, what will the exposure rate be if the same radiographer moves to a position 4 feet from the x-ray tube?

3. If a radiographer stands 5 m from an x-ray tube and is subject to an exposure rate of 4 mR/hr, what will the exposure rate be if the same radiographer moves to a position 10 m from the x-ray tube?

4. If a radiographer stands 1 m from an x-ray tube and is subject to an exposure rate of 7 mR/hr, what will the exposure rate be if the same radiographer moves to a position 2 m from the x-ray tube?

Chapter **9** Protection of Imaging Personnel During Diagnostic X-Ray Procedures

5. If a radiographer stands 6 feet from an x-ray tube and is subject to an exposure rate of 6 mR/hr, what will the exposure rate be if the same radiographer moves to a position 12 feet from the x-ray tube?

6. If a radiographer stands 2 m from an x-ray tube and is subject to an exposure rate of 6 mR/hr, what will the exposure rate be if the same radiographer moves to a position 6 m from the x-ray tube?

The ISL also implies that if a radiographer moves closer to a source of radiation, radiation exposure to the radiographer drastically increases.

Example: If a radiographer stands 1 foot from an x-ray source instead of 6 feet, the radiographer's exposure increases by a factor of $(6/3)^2 = 4$

$$6 \div 3 = 2$$

$$2 \times 2 = 4$$

7. If a radiographer stands 5 m from an x-ray source instead of 10 m, the radiographer's exposure increases by a factor of _____.

8. If a radiographer stands 4 feet from an x-ray source instead of 12 feet, the radiographer's exposure increases by a factor of _____.

9. If a radiographer stands 1 m from an x-ray source instead of 4 m, the radiographer's radiation exposure increases by a factor of _____.

10. If a radiographer stands 2 feet from an x-ray source instead of 8 feet, the radiographer's radiation exposure increases by a factor of _____.

POST TEST

The student should take this test after reading Chapter 9, finishing all accompanying textbook and workbook exercises, and completing any additional activities required by the course instructor. The student should complete the post test with a score of 90% or higher before advancing to the next chapter. (Each of the following 20 questions or blanks is worth 5 points.) Score = _____ %

1. What is the most effective means of protection from ionizing radiation?

_____

2. Most health care facilities have policies for protecting pregnant personnel from radiation. Under these policies an imaging professional who becomes pregnant first informs her supervisor. After this voluntary _____ has been made, the health care facility officially recognizes the pregnancy.

3. Define the term *genetically significant dose.*

_____

_____

4. What poses the greatest occupational hazard for the radiographer in diagnostic radiology?

_____

5. Protective lead aprons and shielded barriers function as _____ shields for diagnostic imaging personnel.

6. State the ISL.

_____

7. Radiographers and nonoccupationally exposed individuals should never stand in the useful beam to _____ a patient during a radiographic procedure.

8. What are the three basic principles of radiation protection?

_____

9. Primary protective barriers are located
   A. At a 45-degree angle to the undeflected line of travel of the x-ray beam
   B. At a 60-degree angle to the undeflected line of travel of the x-ray beam
   C. Parallel to the undeflected line of travel of the x-ray beam
   D. Perpendicular to the undeflected line of travel of the x-ray beam

10. A neck and thyroid shield can guard the thyroid area of occupationally exposed people during general fluoroscopy and x-ray special procedures. It should be
    A. 1-mm lead equivalent
    B. 0.5-mm lead equivalent
    C. 0.25-mm lead equivalent
    D. 0.1-mm lead equivalent

11. For most mobile radiographic units that are not remote controlled, the cord leading to the exposure switch must be long enough to permit the radiographer to stand at least _____ from the patient, the x-ray tube, and the useful beam.
    A. 3 feet
    B. 6 feet
    C. 9 feet
    D. 12 feet

12. During high-level-control fluoroscopic interventional procedures, _____ should be kept so that the cumulative fluoroscopic exposure time may be determined.

13. Occupancy factor, workload, and use factor must be considered when determining _____ requirements for a protective barrier.

14. A spot film device protective curtain, or sliding panel, of a minimum thickness of 0.25-mm lead equivalent normally should be positioned between the fluoroscopist and the patient to intercept _____ radiation above the table top.

15. If a radiographer stands 3 m from an x-ray tube and is subject to an exposure rate of 10 mR/hr, what will the exposure rate be if the same radiographer moves to a position 6 m from the x-ray tube?

_____

16. What type of protective barrier is needed to protect personnel against scatter and leakage radiation?

_____

17. If the image intensifier of a mobile C-arm fluoroscope is positioned as close to the _____ as possible, the required fluoroscopic x-ray beam intensify is minimized.

18. What does the NCRP currently recommend as an annual EqD limit to localized skin and hands?

_____

19. Methods and techniques that reduce patient exposure also reduce exposure for the

_____.

20. It is imperative that the EqD to the embryo-fetus from occupational exposure of the mother not exceed the NCRP-recommended monthly EqD limit of _____ mSv (_____ rem) or a limit of 5 Sv (0.5 rem) during the entire pregnancy.

10 Radiation Monitoring

Chapter 10 covers radiation monitoring, both personnel monitoring and area monitoring. Personnel exposure must be monitored to ensure that occupational radiation exposure levels are kept well below the annual effective dose (EfD) limit. Radiation survey instruments are area monitoring devices that detect and measure radiation. Radiographers and other occupationally exposed individuals must be aware of the various personnel and area radiation exposure monitoring devices and their functions.

CHAPTER HIGHLIGHTS

- Personnel monitoring ensures that occupational radiation exposure levels are kept well below the annual EfD limit.
  - Personnel monitoring is required whenever radiation workers are likely to risk receiving 10% or more of the annual occupational EfD limit of 50 mSv (5 rem) in any single year.
  - To keep radiation exposure as low as reasonably achievable (ALARA), most health care facilities issue dosimeter devices when personnel might receive about 1% of the annual occupational EfD limit (i.e., approximately 0.5 mSv [50 mrem]) in any month.
  - Personnel dosimeters allow assessment of the working habits and conditions of diagnostic imaging personnel over a designated period.
  - A radiation worker should wear a personnel monitoring device at collar level during routine radiographic procedures to approximate the maximum radiation dose to the thyroid, head, and neck.
  - During high-level radiation procedures, imaging professionals should wear a protective lead apron; the dosimeter should be worn outside the garment at collar level to provide a reading of the approximate equivalent dose to the thyroid and eyes.
  - Two personnel dosimeters may be worn during special radiographic procedures. The primary dosimeter is worn outside the lead apron at collar level; a second dosimeter is worn beneath the apron at waist level to monitor the approximate equivalent dose to the lower body trunk.
  - Pregnant radiation workers should wear a second dosimeter to monitor the abdomen.

- Under certain conditions thermoluminescent dosimeter (TLD) ring badges are worn to monitor and determine the equivalent dose to the hands when they are near the primary beam.
- Health care facilities must maintain a record of exposure, as measured by personnel dosimeters, as part of each radiation worker's employment record.
- In general, personnel dosimeters must be portable, durable, and cost-efficient.
- Four types of personnel monitoring devices are available: film badges, optically stimulated luminescence (OSL) dosimeters, pocket ionization chambers, and TLDs.
- To meet state and federal regulations, each health care facility must accurately record and maintain the results of personnel monitoring programs.
- The radiation safety officer (RSO) in a health care facility receives and reviews personnel monitoring reports to assess compliance with ALARA guidelines.
- Monitoring reports list the deep, eye, and shallow occupational exposure of each person wearing the device in the facility, as measured by the exposed monitors.
- Radiation survey instruments are used to perform area monitoring.
  - The detection system indicates the presence or absence of radiation, whereas the dosimeter system measures only cumulative radiation intensity.
  - Radiation survey instruments for area monitoring must be durable and easy to carry, able to detect all common types of ionizing radiation, and unaffected by the energy of the radiation or the direction of the incident radiation.
  - Three types of gas-filled radiation survey instruments are the ionization chamber–type survey meter (cutie pie), the proportional counter, and the Geiger-Muller (G-M) detector.
  - Radiographic and fluoroscopic units can be calibrated with ionization chambers. When an ionization chamber is used for this purpose, it is connected to an electrometer, which can measure tiny electrical currents with a high degree of precision and accuracy.

131

Exercise 1—Crossword Puzzle

Use the clues to complete the crossword puzzle.

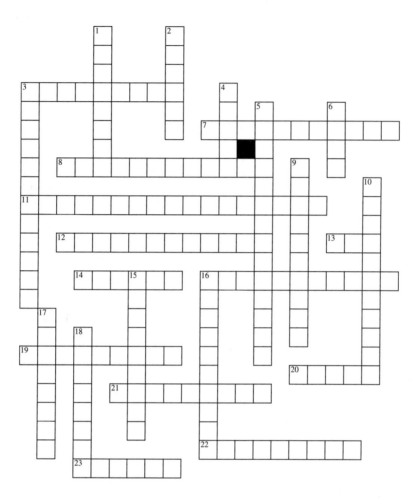

Down

1. A record of this should become part of the employment record of all radiation workers.
2. During routine x-ray procedures, when a protective apron is not being worn, a personnel dosimeter should be worn at this level on the front of the body. all radiation workers.
3. Type of counters not used in diagnostic imaging.
4. What the meter in an ionization chamber-type survey meter does without adequate warm-up time.
5. A graph or curve that represents the response of an image receptor to some probe.
6. Range of radiation exposure measured by a cutie pie within a few seconds.
9. This is recommended for any person occupationally exposed regularly to ionizing radiation.

10. Area where higher occupational exposure can be received.
15. Type of legal record of personnel exposure obtained by a monitoring company reporting badge exposure.
16. Columns on a radiation dosimetry report that provide a continuous audit of actual absorbed radiation equivalent dose.
17. Outside influence that should not affect the performance of a radiation monitor worn by an occupationally exposed person.
18. What exposure monitoring of personnel is whenever radiation workers are likely to risk receiving 10% or more of the annual occupational effective dose limit in any single year.

Across

3. Type of dosimeter worn to monitor exposure.
7. A desirable characteristic for a personnel dosimeter.
8. A device that measures electrical charge.
11. The readout process destroys the stored information in this personnel dosimeter.
12. Word represented by "L" in OSL.
13. Number of months an OSL dosimeter commonly is worn.
14. Metal of which a filter in a film badge is made.
16. What G-M detector tubes tend to lose over time.
19. Type of readout obtained when a pocket ionization chamber is used.

20. If a radiographer wearing a film badge stands too close to a patient during an exposure, this is how the image of the filters in the film badge will appear after the film is developed.
21. Pregnant diagnostic imaging personnel should be issued a 2nd monitoring device to record the radiation dose to the abdomen, during this period of time.
22. Type of dosimeter that a TLD ring badge is.
23. What radiation interacting with the film in a badge causes the film to do once it is developed.

Exercise 2—Matching

Match the following terms with their definitions or associated phrases.

1. _____ personnel dosimeter

2. _____ personnel monitoring report

3. _____ radiation survey instruments

4. _____ OSL

5. _____ second personnel monitoring device
6. _____ Geiger-Müller detector

7. _____ control badge

8. _____ proportional counter

9. _____ optical density
10. _____ ionization chamber connected to an electrometer

11. _____ glow curve

12. _____ check source

13. _____ aluminum oxide (Al_2O_3) detector

14. _____ radiation-dosimetry film

15. _____ exposure monitoring of personnel

16. _____ densitometer

17. _____ pocket dosimeter

18. _____ TLD analyzer
19. _____ ionization chamber–type survey meter

A. The intensity of light transmitted through a given area of the medical imaging film

B. Serves as a basis of comparison with the remaining badges after they have been returned to the monitoring company for processing

C. Device for monitoring occupational exposure that contains an Al_2O_3 detector

D. Resembles an ordinary fountain pen but contains a thimble ionization chamber that measures radiation exposure

E. Cutie pie

F. Contains LiF powder or chips, which function as a sensing material

G. Measures the amount of ionizing radiation to which a TLD badge has been exposed

H. Worn by a pregnant radiographer to monitor the equivalent dose to the embryo-fetus

I. Used to calibrate radiographic and fluoroscopic units

J. Economical type of personnel monitoring device that records whole-body radiation exposure accumulated at a low rate over a long period

K. Provides an indication of the working habits and working conditions of diagnostic imaging personnel

L. Area monitoring device that detects and measures radiation

M. Lists the deep, eye, and shallow occupational exposures of each person in a health care facility as measured by the exposed monitor

N. Device with an audible system that alerts the operator to the presence of ionizing radiation

O. Generally used in laboratories to detect alpha and beta radiation and small amounts of other types of low-level radioactive contamination

P. Radiographic film in a film badge that is sensitive to doses ranging from as low as 0.1 mSv (10 mrem) to as high as 5000 mSv (500 rem)

Q. An instrument that can be used to determine the amount of radiation to which a film badge dosimeter has been exposed

R. Sensing material found in OSL dosimeters

S. Sensing material found in TLDs

Chapter **10** **Radiation Monitoring**

20. _____ TLD

21. _____ film badge

22. _____ lithium fluoride (LiF)

23. _____ ALARA policy

24. _____ fluoroscopy and special procedures

25. _____ TLD ring badge

T. Extremity monitor worn under certain conditions to monitor and determine the equivalent dose to the hands when they are near the primary beam

U. Required whenever radiation workers are likely to risk receiving 10% or more of the annual EfD limit of 50 mSv (5 rem) in any single year

V. Areas of diagnostic radiology that produce the highest occupational radiation exposure for diagnostic imaging personnel

W. A weak, long-lived radioisotope located on the external surface of a G-M detector that is used to verify the daily consistency of the unit

X. Keeping radiation exposure to personnel as low as reasonably achievable

Y. Laser readout of an OSL dosimeter

Exercise 3—Multiple Choice

Select the answer that best completes the following questions or statements.

1. In keeping with the ALARA concept, *most* health care facilities issue personnel dosimetry devices when personnel might receive about _____ of the annual occupational EfD limit in any 1 month.
   A. 25%
   B. 10%
   C. 5%
   D. 1%

2. The detection system of a radiation survey instrument does which of the following?
   A. It measures only cumulative radiation intensity.
   B. It indicates the presence of radiation.
   C. It counts uncharged particles.
   D. A and B

3. Diagnostic imaging personnel should wear a personnel dosimeter during routine operations in an imaging facility because the device provides:
   1. An indication of an individual's working habits
   2. An indication of working conditions in the facility
   3. A way for the employer to determine if radiation workers are actively engaged in performing a specific number of x-ray procedures during a given period
   A. 1 and 2 only
   B. 1 and 3 only
   C. 2 and 3 only
   D. 1, 2, and 3

4. The image densities cast by the filters in the film badge permit which of the following?
   A. Determination of the percentage of visible light emission
   B. Reuse of the radiographic film in the badge
   C. Estimation of the energy of the radiation reaching the badge
   D. Determination of the electrical discharge of the device

5. Which of the following personnel dosimeters allows a radiation worker to determine exposure received as soon as a specific radiologic procedure is completed?
   A. Film badge
   B. OSL dosimeter
   C. Pocket dosimeter
   D. TLD

6. Which of the following instruments should be used in a laboratory to detect alpha and beta radiation and small amounts of other types of low-level radioactive contamination?
   A. Ionization chamber-type survey meter
   B. Proportional counter
   C. G-M detector
   D. Pocket ionization chamber

7. Which of the following devices is used to measure the visible light emitted by the sensing material contained in the TLD *after* exposure to ionizing radiation and heating?
   A. Densitometer
   B. Laser
   C. Photomultiplier tube
   D. Sensitometer

8. In a health care facility, a radiographer's deep, eye, and shallow occupational exposures, as measured by an exposure monitor, may be found on the
   A. Compliance report
   B. Quality assurance report
   C. Personnel monitoring report
   D. Worker's yearly evaluation

9. When the negatively and positively charged electrodes in the pocket ionizing chamber are exposed to ionizing radiation, the mechanism does which of the following?
   A. It charges in direct proportion to the amount of radiation to which it has been exposed
   B. It discharges in direct proportion to the amount of radiation to which it has been exposed
   C. It heats the central electrode
   D. It heats the quartz fiber indicator

10. A densitometer is used to measure which of the following?
   A. The density on the processed radiographic film from a film badge
   B. The light emitted from sensing material of the TLD after exposure
   C. The luminescence from an OSL dosimeter
   D. Freed electrons and discharged electricity from all personnel dosimeters

11. Radiation survey instruments measure which of the following?
   1. The total quantity of electrical charge resulting from ionization of the gas
   2. The rate at which an electrical charge is produced
   3. Luminescence
   A. 1 and 2 only
   B. 1 and 3 only
   C. 2 and 3 only
   D. 1, 2, and 3

12. What do ionization chamber–type survey meters, proportional counters, and G-M detectors have in common?
   A. They measure x-radiation and beta radiation only
   B. They can be used to calibrate radiographic and fluoroscopic x-ray equipment
   C. They are used to measure the radiation dose received outside protective barriers
   D. Each contains a gas-filled chamber

13. Exposure monitoring of personnel is required whenever radiation workers are likely to risk receiving _____ of the annual occupational EfD limit of 50 mSv (5 rem) in any single year.
   A. 1% or less
   B. 5% or less
   C. 7% or less
   D. 10% or less

14. Which of the following are disadvantages of using a TLD as a personnel monitoring device?
   1. Only one readout may be obtained.
   2. A readout or readouts can be lost if the readout procedure is not carefully conducted.
   3. The initial cost is higher than that for a film badge service.
   A. 1 only
   B. 2 only
   C. 3 only
   D. 1, 2, and 3

15. Before a pocket dosimeter is used to record radiation exposure, the quartz fiber indicator of the transparent reading scale should indicate which of the following?
   A. Zero (0)
   B. 100 mR
   C. 150 mR
   D. 200 mR

16. The OSL dosimeter uses
   A. An Al_2O_3 detector
   B. LiF as a sensing material
   C. A miniature ionization chamber as a detector
   D. Radiation dosimetry film as a detector

17. A pocket ionization chamber resembles
   A. A banana
   B. A compass
   C. An ordinary fountain pen
   D. A ruler

18. Monitoring companies send control badges to health care facilities along with each batch of badges. The control badges should be
   A. Given as monitors to radiographers who lose their original badge
   B. Given as a second monitor to pregnant personnel
   C. Given as monitors to radiographers working in the operating room
   D. Kept in a radiation-free area in the imaging facility

19. Badge readings that exceed a trigger level set by the health care facility are investigated to
   A. Ascertain the cause of the reading
   B. Determine whether wearing the badge was actually necessary
   C. Find grounds to fire the radiographer
   D. Increase the workload of the RSO to justify his or her position

20. The TLD readout process
   A. Destroys the information stored in the TLD
   B. Saves the information stored in the TLD for future use
   C. Places the information in a computer
   D. Duplicates the stored information and sends a written report directly to the radiographer

21. An ionization chamber–type survey meter is also referred to as a
    A. Cutie pie
    B. Flux capacitor
    C. Little rascal
    D. Jack in a box

22. The increased sensitivity of the OSL dosimeter makes it ideal for monitoring employees working in low-radiation environments and for
    A. Area monitoring of radioisotope storage facilities
    B. Monitoring of patients with a radioactive implant
    C. Monitoring of pregnant workers
    D. General patient monitoring

23. The RSO in a health care facility receives and reviews personnel monitoring reports to
    A. Assess compliance with ALARA guidelines
    B. Assess compliance with National Academy of Sciences guidelines
    C. Gather information to compile a press report
    D. Meet guidelines established by the Health Insurance Portability and Accountability Act (HIPPA)

24. Wearing a personnel dosimeter in a consistent location is the responsibility of the
    A. RSO
    B. Manager or director of the imaging department
    C. Chief radiologist
    D. Individual wearing the device

25. Upon termination of employment, a radiographer should receive a copy of
    A. All personal health care records kept by the employer
    B. The occupational exposure report
    C. All employment records
    D. Incident reports in which the radiographer was involved

Exercise 4—True or False

Circle *T* if the statement listed below is true; circle *F* if the statement is false.

1. T F Personnel dosimeters protect the wearer from exposure to ionizing radiation.

2. T F Wearing a personnel dosimeter in a consistent location is the responsibility of the individual wearing the device.

3. T F During special radiographic procedures, some health care facilities may prefer to have diagnostic imaging personnel wear two monitoring devices.

4. T F Cost is not a factor for health care facilities in selecting personnel dosimeters.

5. T F The film holder of a film badge dosimeter should be made of a plastic material of a high atomic number to filter low-energy x-radiation, gamma radiation, and beta radiation.

6. T F An ionization chamber–type survey meter cannot be used to measure exposures produced by typical diagnostic procedures because the exposure times are too long to permit the meter to respond.

7. T F A disadvantage of the OSL dosimeter is that occupational exposure cannot be established on the day of occurrence because the badge must be shipped to the monitoring company for reading and exposure determination.

8. T F Pocket ionization chambers require a special charging unit.

9. T F All radiation survey meters are equally sensitive in the detection of ionizing radiation.

10. T F The ionization survey–type meter is used for radiation protection surveys.

11. T F A film badge dosimeter may be worn for up to 1 year.

12. T F In health care facilities that have a well-structured radiation safety program, personnel monitoring reports are received and reviewed by the RSO.

13. T F A personnel dosimeter must be able to detect and record both small and large exposures consistently and reliably.

14. T F The filters in an OSL dosimeter are made of lead, potassium iodide, and zinc.

15. T F Ionizing radiation causes some of the physical properties of the LiF crystals in the TLD to undergo changes.

16. T F When changing employment, the radiation worker must convey the data pertinent to his or her accumulated permanent equivalent dose to the new employer so that this information can be kept on file.

17. T F Although an OSL dosimeter can work for up to 10 years, it commonly is worn for 2 years.

18. T F Pocket dosimeters provide no permanent legal record of exposure.

19. T F The primary advantage of a pocket ionization chamber is that it can provide an immediate exposure readout for radiation workers

in high exposure areas (e.g., a cardiac catheterization laboratory).

20. T F A TLD can be read numerous times.

21. T F Humidity, pressure, and normal temperature changes do not affect TLDs.

22. T F The G-M detector is likely to saturate or jam when placed in a very high-intensity radiation area, consequently giving a false reading.

23. T F Health care facilities must maintain a record of exposure recorded by personnel dosimeters as part of each radiation worker's employment record.

24. T F Area monitoring can be accomplished through the use of radiation survey instruments.

25. T F The image densities cast by the filters in the film badge allow estimation of the energy of the radiation reaching the badge.

Exercise 5—Fill in the Blank

Fill in the blanks with the word or words that best complete the statements below.

1. When the personnel dosimeter is located at collar level, it provides a reading of approximate equivalent dose to the _____ gland and _____ of the occupationally exposed person.

2. A personnel dosimeter must be able to _____ and _____ both small and large exposures consistently and reliably.

3. Personnel dosimeters include film badges, pocket _____ chambers, _____ _____ luminescence dosimeters, and _____ dosimeters.

4. Because many employees in a health care facility may be required to wear radiation monitors, they should be reasonably _____ to purchase and maintain.

5. A single exposure from a primary beam, such as would result if a radiographer inadvertently left the film badge on a table during an exposure, results in a _____ _____ image of the filters in the badge.

6. The control badge should be kept in a _____ area in an imaging facility.

7. When changing employment, the radiation worker must convey those data pertinent to accumulated permanent _____ dose to the new employer.

8. Badge readings that exceed a _____ level set by the health care facility are investigated to ascertain the cause of the reading.

9. Before use each pocket dosimeter must be _____ to a predetermined voltage so that the quartz fiber indicator shows a _____ reading.

10. Radiation survey instruments must be able to detect all _____ types of ionizing radiation.

11. Radiation survey instruments are not all equally _____ in detecting ionizing radiation.

12. Because the G-M detector allows for rapid monitoring, it can be used to locate a _____ radioactive source or low-level radioactive _____.

13. Ionization chambers can be used to _____ radiographic and fluoroscopic equipment.

14. Personnel monitoring ensures that _____ _____ radiation exposure levels are kept well below the annual EfD limit.

15. To keep radiation exposure ALARA, most health care facilities issue dosimeter devices when personnel might receive about _____ % of the annual occupational EfD limit in any month, or approximately _____ mSv (____ mrem).

16. Pregnant radiation workers should wear a second _____ to monitor the abdomen.

17. Monitoring reports list the _____, eye, and _____ occupational exposure of each person wearing the device in the facility as measured by the exposed monitor.

18. After a reading has been obtained, TLD crystals can be _____, making the device somewhat _____.

19. _____ badges indicate whether group badges were exposed in transit to or from a health care facility.

20. The OSL dosimeter provides color coding, graphic formats, and _____ location icons to provide identification.

21. The _____ is an instrument that measures occupational exposure by comparing optical densities of exposed film badges' (dosimetry) film.

22. A TLD is not effective as a monitoring device if it is not _____.

137

23. The film badge provides a permanent _____ record of personnel exposure.

24. The OSL dosimeter gives accurate readings as low as 1 mrem for x-rays and gamma ray photons with energies from _____ keV to _____ MeV.

25. All components of an OSL dosimeter are sealed inside a tamper-proof _____ blister packet.

Exercise 6—Labeling

Label the following illustration.

A. Personnel monitoring devices currently available

_____

    1. _____

    2. _____

    3. _____

    4. _____

    5. _____

_____

Exercise 7—Short Answer

Answer the following questions by providing a short answer.

1. What information is provided by personnel dosimeters?

_____

_____

2. List four types of personnel dosimeters that are used to measure individual exposure of the body to ionizing radiation.

_____

_____

3. What does an extremity dosimeter measure?

_____

_____

4. What information does the badge cover of an extremity monitor contain?

_____

_____

5. What is optical density?

_____

_____

6. List three radiation survey instruments that are used for area monitoring.

_____

_____

7. Where are proportional counters used? What do they detect?

_____

_____

8. List some disadvantages of a TLD.

_____

_____

9. What kind of detector is found in an OSL dosimeter?

_____

_____

10. What is the sensitivity range of radiation-dosimetry film?

_____

_____

11. When is exposure monitoring of personnel required?

_____

_____

12. When a protective lead apron is used during fluoroscopy or special procedures, why should the personnel dosimeter be worn outside the apron at collar level on the anterior surface of the body?

_____

_____

13. What do occupational exposure values found on a record of radiation exposure represent?

_____

_____

14. What does the letter "M" indicate when it appears under the current monitoring period or in the cumulative columns of a personnel monitoring report?

_____

_____

15. What must a radiation worker do when changing employment?

_____

_____

Exercise 8—Essay

On a separate sheet of paper, answer the following questions in essay form.

1. Describe the use of a G-M detector as an area radiation survey instrument.

2. Describe the role the RSO fulfills in department safety and in monitoring of radiation exposure.

3. Explain the importance of radiation exposure monitoring for occupationally exposed personnel.

4. Describe the use of the ionization chamber–type survey meter for radiation protection surveys.

5. Describe the evolution of personnel dosimeters used for monitoring of occupational radiation exposure.

POST TEST

The student should take this test after reading Chapter 10, finishing all accompanying textbook and workbook exercises, and completing any additional activities required by the course instructor. The student should complete the post test with a score of 90% or higher before advancing to the next chapter. (Each of the following 20 questions or blanks is worth 5 points.) Score = _____ %

1. Some means of monitoring personnel must be used to ensure that occupational radiation exposure levels are kept well below the annual _____ dose limit.

2. Define the term *optically stimulated luminescence dosimeter.*

_____

_____

3. How can the working habits and conditions of diagnostic imaging personnel be assessed over a designated period?

_____

_____

4. To meet state and federal regulations, _____ from personnel monitoring programs must be recorded accurately and maintained by each health care facility.

5. Where should a radiation worker wear a personnel monitoring device during routine radiographic procedures to approximate the maximum radiation dose to the thyroid, head, and neck?

_____

6. Which of the following devices are used for personnel monitoring?
   1. OSL dosimeter
   2. TLD
   3. Ionization chamber–type survey meter (cutie pie)
   A. 1 and 2 only
   B. 1 and 3 only
   C. 2 and 3 only
   D. 1, 2, and 3

7. LiF functions as the sensing material in which of the following devices?
   A. Film badge
   B. OSL dosimeter
   C. Pocket dosimeter
   D. TLD

8. In a health care facility, where can a radiographer's deep, eye, and shallow occupational exposure as measured by an exposed monitor be found?

_____

_____

9. What instrument should be used to locate a lost radioactive source or to detect low-level radioactive contamination?

_____

10. Before a pocket dosimeter is used to record radiation exposure, the quartz fiber indicator of the transparent reading scale should indicate _____.

11. In addition to a primary personnel dosimeter, pregnant imaging personnel should be issued a second monitoring device to record the radiation dose to the _____ during gestation to provide an estimate of the equivalent dose to the embryo-fetus.

12. When radiation workers change employment, what must they convey to the new employer?

_____

_____

13. Radiation survey instruments are area monitoring devices that detect and _____ radiation.

14. Health care facilities must maintain a record of exposure recorded by personnel dosimeters as part of each radiation worker's _____ record.

15. When are radiation workers required to wear personnel monitoring devices?

_____

_____

16. It is recommended that an extremity dosimeter, or TLD ring badge, be worn by an imaging professional as a second monitor whenever procedures are performed that require the hands to be near the _____ x-ray beam.

17. In a health care facility who generally receives and reviews personnel monitoring reports?

_____

18. Although an OSL dosimeter can be worn for up to 1 year, it commonly is worn for _____ months.

19. What is used to calibrate radiographic and fluoroscopic x-ray equipment?

_____

20. In diagnostic imaging, the increased sensitivity of the OSL dosimeter makes it ideal for monitoring employees working in low-radiation environments and for _____ workers.

11 Radioisotopes and Radiation Protection

Chapter 11 covers radioisotopes and radiation protection. This chapter briefly discusses the use of radioisotopes for both diagnostic and therapeutic medical procedures, as well as some relevant radiation issues. It also focuses on the use of radiation as a terrorist weapon and includes some fundamental principles of dealing with radioactive contamination in the health care setting.

CHAPTER HIGHLIGHTS

- *Isotopes* are atoms that have the same number of protons in the nucleus but different numbers of neutrons.
  - Some nuclei of isotopes have too many neutrons or too many protons.
  - Radioactive isotopes spontaneously undergo changes, or transformations, to rectify their unstable arrangements.
- Rapidly dividing cells that are well oxygenated are very radiosensitive.
  - When cells are radiosensitive, cancerous growths or tumors can be eliminated or at least controlled by irradiation of the area containing the growth.
- Therapeutic isotopes may be characterized by relatively long half-lives.
- Fast electrons are known as *beta radiation.*
- Gamma rays and x-ray photons differ only in their point of origin.
- Iodine-125 (^{125}I) decays with a half-life of 59.4 days by a process called *electron capture.*
- Distance and time constitute the most practical radiation protection for patients having therapeutic prostate seed implants.
- The radioactive isotope Strontium-89 (^{89}Sr) is a bone seeker.
- A *neutrino* is a particle that has negligible mass and no electric charge but carries away any excess energy from the nucleus of the atom.
- During administration of iodine-131 (^{131}I) to treat a hospitalized patient for thyroid cancer, a large (up to 1 inch thick) rolling lead shield can be positioned between the patient and any attending personnel for protection.
- Diagnostic techniques in nuclear medicine typically involve the use of short-lived radioisotopes as radioactive tracers.
  - Technetium-99m (^{99m}Tc) is the radioisotope most frequently used in nuclear medicine.
- Positron emission tomography (PET) makes use of annihilation radiation events.
  - When annihilation occurs, the positron and electron interact destructively and annihilate each other. Their respective masses convert into energy, which is carried off by two photons emerging from the annihilation site in opposite directions, each with a kinetic energy of 511 keV.
  - Fluorine-18 (^{18}F) is the most important isotope used for PET scanning.
- PET is an important imaging modality because it allows examination of the metabolic processes in the body.
- Fluorodeoxyglucose (FDG) is a radioactive tracer that is taken up or metabolized by cancerous cells; it also reveals the locations of these cells through its positron emission decay and subsequent generation of oppositely traveling annihilation photons.
- A PET/CT scanner can detect abnormally high regions of glucose metabolism, yielding evidence of metastasis to other body areas, and can provide detailed information about the location and size of these lesions or growths.
- Positron emission results in the production of high-energy radiation, therefore the design of a PET/CT imaging suite involves significant radiation safety concerns.
- Most hospitals have radiation emergency plans for handling emergencies involving radioactive contamination.
- A radioactive dispersal device, or *dirty bomb,* is a radioactive source mixed with conventional explosives; the actual long-term health effects of these devices are most likely to be minimal.
  - If radioactive material from a dirty bomb remains in a small area, few people may be affected. On the other hand, if enough explosives are used to spread the radioactive material over a broad area, the radioactivity will be diluted and may not be much higher than background levels.
  - If a dirty bomb exploded with the same force as the explosion at Chernobyl, the actual number of radiation injuries could be quite small.
- The United States currently has emergency responders who are prepared and equipped to monitor and assess personnel exposure on site at an emergency.
  - After explosion of a dirty bomb, externally contaminated individuals can be decontaminated by removing contaminated clothing and immersion in a shower.
  - Geiger-Müller (GM) detectors can be used by trained emergency personnel to monitor contamination levels.
  - During an emergency situation, individuals engaged in nonlifesaving activities work under a dose limit of 50 mSv (5 rem) per event; those performing lifesaving activities have a dose limit of 250 mSv (25 rem).
  - If surface contamination is suspected, emergency personnel should protect themselves by wearing gowns, masks, and gloves while working with the patient.
  - Handling of patients with internal contamination varies, depending on the clinical and radiologic form of contamination. Strategies may include dilution and blocking of absorption in the gastrointestinal tract. Potassium iodide can be administered to block uptake of radioactive iodine in the thyroid gland.

Exercise 1—Crossword Puzzle

Use the clues to complete the crossword puzzle.

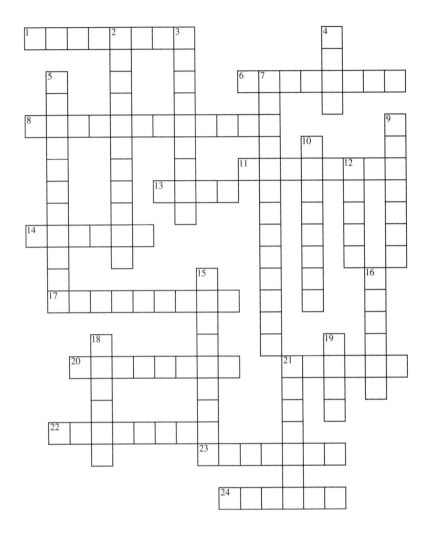

Down

2. Type of isotopes that are characterized by relatively long half-lives.
3. Element that has the same chemical properties as calcium.
4. Type of radiation that fast electrons are.
5. Where radioactive tablets dissolve in the human body.
7. Used in Nuclear Medicine to detect the spread of cancer into bone.
9. Type of energy possessed by two photons emerging from an annihilation site.
10. A well-designed PET-CT scanning facility will take good advantage of this powerful radiation protection tool.
12. If a wound contains radioactive material, this procedure is usually sufficient to decontaminate the

area to allow medical personnel to provide medical attention.
15. What it may be to monitor all workers involved in a radiation emergency.
16. One item that personnel should wear when working with a patient who has received radioactive surface contamination.
18. Type of public concern that the explosion of a dirty bomb will become.
19. Level of energy that annihilation photons emanating in all directions from the patient having a PET/CT scan study possess.
21. Form of ordinary sugar that the radioactive tracer FDG is similar to in chemical behavior.

Chapter **11** **Radioisotopes and Radiation Protection**

Across

1. For a patient suffering from radiation sickness, the aspect that medical management should be geared to treat during the first 48 hours after exposure.
6. Gland in which Iodine-125 seeds may be implanted for therapeutic purposes.
8. Condition of clothing that would need to be removed during the process of radioactive decontamination.
11. Positively charged electron.
13. After an explosion of a dirty bomb, this radioactive material will contaminate some individuals.
14. Point where gamma rays and x-rays differ.

17. Type of processes in the human body examined by Positron Emission Tomography.
20. Table that lists the elements.
21. Counter that is used to monitor radioactive contamination.
22. Surface contamination.
23. Gland where sodium iodide (^{123}I) will preferentially concentrate.
24. Type of significant radiation concerns that PET/CT imaging suites involve.

Exercise 2—Matching

Match the following terms with their definitions or associated phrases.

1. _____ PET/CT scanner

2. _____ radiation emergency plan
3. _____ beta decay

4. _____ decontamination

5. _____ Environmental Protection Agency (EPA)
6. _____ half-value layer (HVL)

7. _____ radioisotopes

8. _____ radioactive contamination

9. _____ ^{18}F

10. _____ surface contamination

11. _____ neutrino

12. _____ annihilation radiation

13. _____ proton

14. _____ nuclear medicine
15. _____ isotopes

16. _____ FDG

17. _____ electron capture
18. _____ neutron

A. An electrically neutral particle that is believed to have almost negligible mass
B. Dirty bomb
C. Process through which an inner shell electron is captured by one of the nuclear protons; the two then combine to produce a neutron, thereby creating a different element
D. Atoms that have the same number of protons in the nucleus but different numbers of neutrons
E. Byproduct of the pair production interaction
F. Radioactive tracer compound similar in chemical behavior to ordinary glucose; it therefore is taken up or metabolized by cancerous cells, revealing their location through its radioactive decay process
G. Modality that uses ionizing radiation for the treatment of disease, namely, cancer
H. Isotopes of a particular element that are unstable because of their neutron-proton configuration
I. Modality that produces axial images by making use of annihilation radiation that is initiated by positron radioactive decay of the nucleus of an unstable atom
J. Removal of radioactive material from an area or from clothing or a person
K. Process by which a nucleus relieves an instability through conversion of a neutron to a proton, and an electron, and a neutrino, with emission of the electron and the neutrino
L. Branch of medicine that uses radioisotopes to study organ function, to detect the spread of cancer into bone, and to treat certain types of disease
M. U.S. government agency that facilitates the development and enforcement of regulations controlling radiation in the environment; it sets limits for radioactive contamination that assume that a 1 in 10,000 risk of causing a fatal cancer is unacceptable
N. Radioactive isotope used for PET scanning
O. Radioactive material that is attached to or associated with dust particles or is in liquid form on various surfaces
P. Process by which a computer-reconstructed transverse (or axial) image of a patient is created by an x-ray tube detector assembly rotating 360 degrees about a specific part of the body
Q. Energy of motion
R. A device that detects individual radioactive particles or photons and that also serves as the primary radiation survey instrument for area monitoring in nuclear medicine facilities

19. _____ computed axial tomography (CAT)

S. A unit that is physically joined in a tandem configuration with a CAT scanner to produce a one-joint imaging device; using FDG F-18, it can detect abnormally high regions of glucose metabolism, which are evidence of the spread of cancer or of metastatic disease in other body areas; it also provides detailed information about the location and size of these lesions or growths

20. _____ positron

T. The thickness of a designated absorber required to reduce the intensity of the primary beam by 50% of its initial value

21. _____ Geiger-Müller (G-M) detector

U. A positively charged electron, which is a form of antimatter

22. _____ kinetic energy

V. A plan hospitals can implement for handling emergencies involving radioactive contamination

23. _____ radiation therapy

W. External contamination of the skin or clothing with radioactive material

24. _____ PET

X. An electrically neutral particle found in the nucleus of the atom; one of the fundamental constituents of the atom

25. _____ radioactive dispersal device

Y. One of the three main constituents of an atom, it carries a positive electrical charge

Exercise 3—Multiple Choice

Select the answer that best completes the following questions or statements.

1. Isotopes are atoms that have the *same* number of _____ in the nucleus but *different* numbers of _____.
   A. electrons, protons
   B. neutrons, electrons
   C. protons, neutrons
   D. protons, neutrinos

2. Which two terms are synonymous?
   A. X-rays and gamma rays
   B. Alpha rays and beta rays
   C. Fast electrons and beta rays
   D. Neutrons and neutrinos

3. Which of the following radioisotopes used in radiation therapy is considered a bone seeker?
   A. ^{125}I
   B. ^{125}Te
   C. ^{131}I
   D. ^{89}Sr

4. A particle that has negligible mass and no electrical charge but that carries away excess energy from the nucleus of the atom is a (an):
   A. Electron
   B. Neutron
   C. Neutrino
   D. Proton

5. The branch of medicine that uses radioisotopes to study organ function, to detect the spread of cancer into bone, and to treat certain types of disease is:
   A. Chemotherapy
   B. Computed radiography
   C. Nuclear medicine
   D. Ultrasonography

6. The radioisotope *most often* used in nuclear medicine diagnostic studies is:
   A. ^{125}I
   B. ^{131}I
   C. ^{89}Sr
   D. ^{99m}Tc

7. PET makes use of what radiation events?
   A. Annihilation radiation
   B. Compton scattering
   C. Photodisintegration
   D. Photoelectric interaction

8. During the process of annihilation, the positron and the electron annihilate each other and their rest masses are converted into energy, which appears in the form of two 511 keV photons, each moving:
   A. At exactly 45-degree angles to each other
   B. In the same direction
   C. In opposite directions
   D. Toward the nucleus of the original atom

9. The isotope *most often* used in PET scanning is:
   A. ^{60}Co
   B. ^{18}F
   C. ^{131}I
   D. ^{89}Sr

10. Positron emitters result in the production of
    A. High-energy radiation
    B. Intermediate-energy radiation
    C. Low-energy radiation
    D. No radiation

11. Most hospitals have _____ for handling emergencies involving radioactive contamination.
    A. No radiation emergency plans
    B. No trained personnel
    C. Radiation emergency plans and trained personnel
    D. A and B

12. A 1 in 10,000 probability of causing a fatal cancer corresponds to an effective dose of approximately
    A. 1 mSv (100 rem)
    B. 2 mSv (200 rem)
    C. 3 mSv (300 rem)
    D. 5 mSv (500 rem)

13. For exposures localized to *specific* regions of the body, medical management involves
    1. Prevention of infection
    2. Control of pain
    3. Possibly skin grafts
    A. 1 and 2 only
    B. 1 and 3 only
    C. 2 and 3 only
    D. 1, 2, and 3

14. The physical half-life of ^{18}F is
    A. 10 minutes
    B. 110 minutes
    C. 10 years
    D. 110 years

15. ^{125}I is an unstable isotope of the element iodine with
    A. 73 protons and 102 neutrons
    B. 102 protons and 73 neutrons
    C. 53 protons and 72 neutrons
    D. 72 protons and 53 neutrons

16. The design of a PET/CT imaging suite involves
    A. No radiation safety concerns
    B. Minimal radiation safety concerns
    C. Moderate radiation safety concerns
    D. Significant radiation safety concerns

17. Each _____ nuclear transformation by positron decay yields two highly penetrating 511 keV photons.
    A. ^{18}Cl
    B. ^{18}F
    C. ^{18}I
    D. ^{18}Sr

18. In beta decay a neutron transforms itself into a combination of
    A. A positron and an alpha particle
    B. A positron and a negatron
    C. A proton and an energetic electron
    D. A proton and an alpha particle

19. Radioactive ^{89}Sr is a
    A. Bone evader
    B. Bone demineralizer
    C. Bone mineralizer
    D. Bone seeker

20. Fast electrons are
    A. Alpha radiation
    B. Beta radiation
    C. Gamma radiation
    D. X-radiation

21. A neutrino is a particle that has a _____ mass and _____ electrical charge but carries away any excess energy from the nucleus of the atom.
    A. significant, positive
    B. significant, negative
    C. negligible, no
    D. negligible, positive

22. Gamma rays and x-ray photons only differ in their
    A. Wavelength
    B. Position on the electromagnetic spectrum
    C. Point of origin
    D. Energy and frequency

23. If a dirty bomb exploded with the same force as the explosion at the Chernobyl nuclear power station in 1986, the actual number of injuries attributed to radiation exposure could be
    A. Catastrophic
    B. Enormous
    C. Quite small
    D. Nonexistent

24. Potassium iodide can be administered to block further uptake of radioactive iodine in the
    A. Gallbladder
    B. Liver
    C. Kidneys
    D. Thyroid gland

25. The thickness of a designated absorber required to reduce the intensity of the primary beam by 50% of its initial value defines
    A. Radioisotope shielding barrier equivalent
    B. Lead apron thickness requirement
    C. HVL
    D. Positron emission

Exercise 4—True or False

Circle *T* if the statement listed below is true; circle *F* if the statement is false.

1. T F ^{125}I is a stable isotope.

2. T F Distance and time are the best radiation safety practices for therapeutic implants such as the ^{125}I seed implant for the prostate gland.

3. T F Hospital rooms for ^{131}I patients usually are isolated and carefully prepared with absorbent cloths to substantially minimize radiation exposure to personnel and visitors from emitted gamma radiation from the patient or from contaminated surfaces.

4. T F In a PET device, annihilation radiation is initiated by the radioactive decay of the nucleus of a stable atom.

5. T F The nucleus of ^{18}F has 18 neutrons.

6. T F The possible use of radiation as a terrorist weapon is of no concern to the general population.

7. T F If radioactive material from a dirty bomb remains is a small area, few people might be affected.

8. T F Because monitoring of all workers involved in a radiation emergency may be difficult, a dose rate criterion often is used.

9. T F The same procedures that control infection are not useful for preventing the spread of radioactive contamination.

10. T F Diagnostic techniques in nuclear medicine typically make use of long-lived radio-isotopes as radioactive tracers.

11. T F ^{131}I is the radioisotope most often used in nuclear medicine.

12. T F ^{89}Sr is a pure beta emitter.

13. T F It is important that a hospital have a radiation emergency plan for handling emergencies involving radioactive contamination.

14. T F In the United States, emergency responders are equipped to monitor and assess personnel exposure on site at an emergency.

15. T F Most hospitals stock cutie pies to monitor radiation contamination levels during an emergency.

16. T F Radiation therapy uses ionizing radiation for the radiologic diagnosis of disease.

17. T F Radioactive contamination may consist of surface, internal (inhaled or ingested), internal wound, or external wound contamination.

18. T F A positron is a normal form of matter.

19. T F ^{123}I undergoes radioactive decay by the process of electron capture, with an average half-life of 13.3 hours.

20. T F ^{99m}Tc is an extremely versatile radioisotope because it can be incorporated into a wide variety of different compounds or biologically active substances, each with a specificity for different tissues or organs.

21. T F Each ^{18}F nuclear transformation by positron decay yields two highly penetrating 511 keV photons, which can be shielded by an ordinary lead apron.

22. T F ^{18}F has a physical half-life of 110 minutes, therefore the patient's degree of radioactivity declines naturally throughout the preparation time, with approximately 25% to 30% lost by the time of scanning.

23. T F The only cases of acute radiation syndrome at Chernobyl were among emergency workers, primarily firemen who worked very near the reactor.

24. T F A dirty bomb is unlikely to cause contamination with so much radioactive material that a victim could not receive medical attention.

25. T F Removal of surface radioactive contamination involves removing the clothing and showering to cleanse the skin.

Exercise 5—Fill in the Blank

Fill in the blanks with the word or words that best complete the statements below.

1. For ^{125}I seed implants, the goal is to deliver 145 Gy to at least _____% of the prostate's volume while limiting the radiation dose as much as possible to _____ structures such as the urethra, bladder, and anterior rectal wall.

2. For cancer patients in whom other methods of treatment have failed and who now have _____ to bone, infusion of ^{89}Sr delivers radiation therapy to those areas.

3. ^{99m}Tc has a half-life of _____ hours and decays by emission from its _____, primarily of gamma ray photons of 140 keV energy.

4. _____ emitters produce high-energy radiation.

5. Every patient who is to have a PET/CT scan requires _____ time.

6. With the attack on the World Trade Center on September 11, 2001, the possibility of the use of other possible terrorist weapons, such as _____, has become a public health concern.

7. A radioactive source mixed with conventional explosives describes a radioactive dispersal device, or _____ _____.

8. Rapidly dividing cells that are well oxygenated are very _____.

9. Fast-moving electrons are called _____ radiation.

10. ^{125}I decays with a 59.4 half-life process called _____ _____.

11. During administration of Iodine-131 (^{131}I) to treat a hospitalized patient for thyroid cancer, a large (up to 1 inch thick) rolling lead shield can be positioned between _____ and any attending personnel for protection.

12. Radioactive isotopes spontaneously undergo changes or transformations to rectify their _____ arrangement.

13. PET makes use of _____ radiation events.

14. PET is an important imaging modality because it can examine _____ processes in the body.

15. _____ counters can be used by trained emergency personnel to monitor radioactive contamination levels.

16. Handling of patients with internal contamination will _____, depending on the clinical and radiologic form of contamination.

17. Clothing that has been contaminated with radioactive material should be placed in a _____ _____ and set aside for later evaluation.

18. ^{125}I patients should significantly limit the duration of close contact <3 feet (1 m) with small children and _____ women for _____ months after the implant procedure.

19. Strontium and _____ are members of the same family of elements in the periodic table.

20. For a patient who has thyroid cancer, it is desirable to strongly irradiate any _____ thyroid tissue not removed by surgery while significantly _____ surrounding tissue and other organs.

21. Hospital rooms for ^{131}I therapy patients usually are _____ and carefully prepared with absorbent cloths to substantially _____ radiation exposure to both personnel and visitors from gamma radiation emitted from the patient or from contaminated surfaces.

22. ^{123}I is a _____ compound.

23. The nucleus of ^{18}F has _____ neutrons.

24. A well-designed PET/CT facility is arranged so that no areas of _____ occupancy are adjacent to a high-energy radiation source.

25. _____ of all radiation workers involved in a radiation emergency may be difficult.

Exercise 6—Labeling

Label the following table.

A. Dose-effect relationship after acute whole-body radiation from gamma rays or x-rays*

Whole-Body Absorbed Dose	Effect
0.05 Gy	No symptoms
1._____	No symptoms, but possible chromosomal aberrations in cultured peripheral-blood lymphocytes
2._____	No symptoms (minor decreases in white blood cell and platelet counts in a few persons)
3._____	Nausea and vomiting in approximately 10 percent of persons within 48 hours after exposure
4._____	Nausea and vomiting in approximately 50% of persons within 24 hr, with marked decreases in white blood cell and platelet counts
5._____	Nausea and vomiting in 90% of persons within 12 hr, and diarrhea in 10% within 8 hr; 50% mortality in the absence of medical treatment
6._____	100% mortality within 30 days due to bone marrow failure in the absence of medical treatment
7._____	Approximate dose that is survivable with the best medical therapy available
8._____	Nausea and vomiting in all persons in less than 5 min; severe gastrointestinal damage; death likely in 2 to 3 wk in the absence of treatment
9._____	Cardiovascular collapse and central nervous system damage, with death in 24 to 72 hr

*Gusev I, Guskova AK, Mettler FA Jr, editors: *Medical management of radiation accidents*, ed 2, Boca Raton, Fla., 2001, CRC Press.

Exercise 7—Short Answer

Answer the following questions by providing a short answer.

1. How are therapeutic isotopes characterized?

_____

_____

2. How does electron capture occur?

_____

_____

3. How does beta decay occur?

_____

_____

4. What type of radioisotopes typically are used in nuclear medicine as radioactive tracers? How do these radio-nuclides work?

_____

_____

5. Why is PET an important imaging modality?

_____

_____

6. What benefit does the radioactive tracer FDG provide in PET imaging?

_____

_____

7. What benefit is obtained by combining PET and CT into one imaging device, called a PET/CT scanner?

_____

_____

8. What event led to the possibility of radiation being used as a terrorist weapon?

_____

_____

9. Why does the EPA set limits for radioactive contamination?

_____

_____

Chapter **11** **Radioisotopes and Radiation Protection**

10. What protective apparel should personnel wear if a patient has surface radioactive contamination?

_____

_____

11. Besides trained emergency personnel, who would be available to assess radioactive contamination in a health care facility during a radiation emergency?

_____

_____

12. How do personnel adhere to normal badge limits during a radiation emergency?

_____

_____

13. Describe the medical management of a patient during the first 48 hours of treatment for acute radiation syndrome.

_____

_____

14. What is annihilation radiation?

_____

_____

15. What is a radioactive dispersal device?

_____

_____

Exercise 8—Essay

On a separate sheet of paper, answer the following questions in essay form.

1. Describe the process of PET/CT scanning.

2. Describe some of the problems that may be encountered in designing shielding for a PET/CT department.

3. Describe the role of a radiologic technologist in a health care facility during a radiation emergency.

4. Describe the radiation protective measures that both physicians and staff members can use when providing medical care to a patient contaminated with radiation (externally/internally).

5. Describe a scenario that involves a radioactive dispersal device (dirty bomb). Include possible health and community consequences and the emergency response to the situation with emphasis on radiation safety.

POST TEST

The student should take this test after reading Chapter 11, finishing all accompanying textbook and workbook exercises, and completing any additional activities required by the course instructor. The student should complete the post test with a score of 90% or higher before advancing to the next chapter. (Each of the following 20 questions or blanks is worth 5 points.) Score = _____ %

1. What U.S. government agency facilitates the development and enforcement of regulations controlling radiation in the environment and sets limits for radioactive contamination that assume that a 1 in 10,000 risk of causing a fatal cancer is unacceptable?

_____

2. Define *radioactive dispersal device.*

_____

_____

3. How are therapeutic radioisotopes characterized?

_____

_____

4. ^{18}F has a physical half-life of
   A. 110 seconds
   B. 110 minutes
   C. 110 hours
   D. 110 years

5. Isotopes are atoms that have the same number of protons in the nucleus but different numbers of _____.

6. _____ dividing cells that are well oxygenated are very radiosensitive.

7. What is a neutrino?

_____

_____

8. After a dirty bomb explosion, how can externally contaminated individuals be decontaminated?

_____

_____

9. Of what radiation events does PET make use?

_____

10. A 1 in 10,000 probability of causing a fatal cancer corresponds to an effective dose of approximately _____ mSv (_____ mrem).

11. A radioactive tracer that is taken up or metabolized by cancerous cells and reveals their locations through its positron emission decay and subsequent generation of oppositely traveling annihilation photons is _____.

12. Diagnostic techniques in nuclear medicine typically make use of _____ radioisotopes as radioactive tracers.

13. During an emergency, under what dose limit are individuals performing lifesaving activities allowed to work?

_____

14. Define the term *electron capture*.

_____

_____

15. In what do positron emitters result?

_____

_____

16. What radiation survey instrument is used by emergency personnel to monitor radioactive contamination?

_____

17. What radioisotope is most often used in nuclear medicine diagnostic studies?

_____

18. What do most hospitals have for handling emergencies involving radioactive contamination?

_____

_____

19. A well-designed PET/CT facility is arranged so that no areas of full occupancy are adjacent to a _____ _____ radiation source.

20. Fast-moving electrons are _____ radiation.

Answer Key

Chapter 1

Exercise 1—Crossword Puzzle

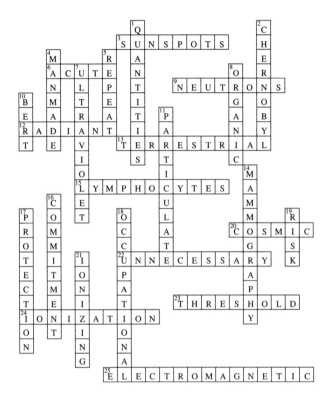

Exercise 2—Matching
1. P	6. A	11. I	16. J	21. L
2. X	7. H	12. E	17. O	22. S
3. F	8. Y	13. T	18. R	23. M
4. C	9. G	14. D	19. N	24. Q
5. K	10. B	15. W	20. U	25. V

Exercise 3—Multiple Choice
1. C	6. C	11. C	16. B	21. D
2. B	7. D	12. D	17. C	22. C
3. C	8. B	13. D	18. D	23. D
4. A	9. B	14. D	19. C	24. B
5. B	10. C	15. B	20. A	25. C

Exercise 4—True or False
1. T
2. T
3. T
4. F (No threshold exists.)
5. F (3 mSv/yr [approximately 300 mrem/yr])
6. T
7. F (They vary.)
8. F (EqD enables the calculation of EfD.)
9. F (They are continuously exposed.)
10. T
11. F (No atmospheric nuclear testing has occurred since 1980.)
12. F (They produce negligible radiation exposure.)
13. T
14. T
15. F (Alpha particles can be absorbed; they are very damaging to radiosensitive epithelial tissue.)
16. F (approximately 0.3 mSv [30 mrem]/yr)
17. T
18. T
19. F (A neutron has approximately the same mass as a proton.)
20. F (a classic example of organic damage)
21. T
22. F (Smokers exposed to high radon levels have a higher risk of lung cancer than do nonsmokers.)
23. F (Solar contribution to the cosmic ray background increases.)
24. T
25. T

Exercise 5—Fill in the Blank
1. radiation dose, dose rates
2. latent period
3. ETHOS Project
4. benefits, far outweigh
5. energy, biologic effects
6. terrestrial
7. Cosmic
8. radionuclides
9. equivalent dose
10. x-ray machines, radiopharmaceuticals
11. safe operation
12. benefits, outweigh, risk
13. ALARA
14. BERT, comparison
15. radon, lung
16. Radionuclides
17. greatest, lowest
18. 600, 60,000
19. 0.0116, 1.16
20. Thyroid
21. justify, responsibility
22. beneficial, destructive
23. 40, molten
24. higher
25. frequencies. wavelengths

153

Exercise 6—Labeling

A.

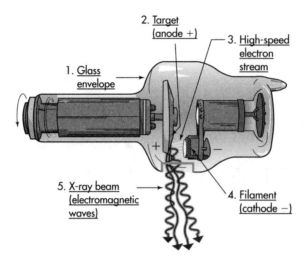

1. Glass envelope
2. Target (anode +)
3. High-speed electron stream
4. Filament (cathode −)
5. X-ray beam (electromagnetic waves)

B.

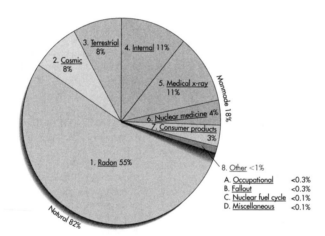

1. Radon 55%
2. Cosmic 8%
3. Terrestrial 8%
4. Internal 11%
5. Medical x-ray 11%
6. Nuclear medicine 4%
7. Consumer products 3%
8. Other <1%
  A. Occupational   <0.3%
  B. Fallout   <0.3%
  C. Nuclear fuel cycle   <0.1%
  D. Miscellaneous   <0.1%

Manmade 18%

Natural 82%

From National Council on Radiation Protection and Measurements (NCRP): *Report No. 93, ionizing radiation exposure of the population of the United States,* Bethesda, MD, 1987, The Council.

C.

Radiation Equivalent Dose and Subsequent Biologic Effects Resulting from Acute Whole Body Exposures*

Radiation Equivalent Dose (EqD)	Subsequent Biologic Effect
1. 0.25 Sv (25 rem)	Blood changes (e.g., measurable hematologic depression, decreases in the number of lymphocytes present in the circulating blood)
2. 1.5 Sv (150 rem)	Nausea, diarrhea
3. 2.0 Sv (200 rem)	Erythema (diffuse redness over an area of skin after irradiation)
4. 2.5 Sv (250 rem)	If dose is to gonads, temporary sterility
5. 3.0 Sv (300 rem)	50% chance of death; lethal dose for 50% of population over 30 days (LD 50/30)
6. 6.0 Sv (600 rem)	Death

*Radiation exposures are delivered to the entire body over a time period of less than a few hours.
Modified from Radiologic health, unit 4, slide 17, Denver, Multi-Media Publishing (slide program).

154

Answer Key

Exercise 7—Short Answer

1. Human beings can exercise greater control over the use of radiant energy by using the knowledge of radiation hazards that has been gained over many years and by employing methods to limit or eliminate those hazards.

2. Radiologic technologists and radiologists can reduce radiation exposure to patients and to themselves by using protective devices whenever possible, by following established procedures, and by selecting technical exposure factors that significantly reduce radiation exposure.

3. Ionizing radiation produces damage while penetrating normal body tissue, primarily by ejecting electrons from the atoms making up the tissues.

4. The amount of energy transferred to electrons by ionizing radiation is the basis of the concept of radiation dose.

5. If excessive cellular damage occurs as a consequence of radiation exposure, the living organism exhibits genetic or somatic changes.

6. Cosmic rays are of extraterrestrial origin. They result from nuclear interactions that have taken place in the sun and other stars.

7. Potassium-40 (^{40}K); carbon-14 (^{14}C); hydrogen-3 (^{3}H, Tritium); and strontium-90 (^{90}Sr)

8. The total annual equivalent dose from fallout cannot be estimated accurately because actual radiation measurements do not exist. The dose commitment may be estimated by using a series of approximations and simplistic models that are subject to considerable speculation.

9. When ionizing radiation is used for the welfare of the patient, the directly realized benefits of the exposure to this radiant energy must far outweigh any slight risk of induction of a radiogenic malignancy or genetic defect.

10. The patient dose for each x-ray procedure varies from one health care facility to another because of the large variety of radiologic equipment and the differences in imaging procedures and the technical skills of individual radiologists and radiographers.

11. Six consequences of ionization in human cells are (1) creation of unstable atoms; (2) production of free electrons; (3) production of low-energy x-ray photons; (4) creation of reactive free radicals capable of producing substances poisonous to the cell; (5) creation of new biologic molecules detrimental to the living cell; and (6) injury to the cell that may manifest itself as abnormal function or loss of function.

12. Nonionizing infrared and ultraviolet radiation actually produces the sensation of heat or the chemical changes that produce suntan and sunburn.

13. The millirem, a subunit of the rem, is equal to $^{1}/_{1000}$ of a rem.

14. Six sources of manmade (artificial) ionizing radiation are (1) consumer products containing radioactive material; (2) air travel; (3) nuclear fuel for generating power; (4) atmospheric fallout from nuclear weapons; (5) nuclear power plant accidents; and (6) medical radiation.

15. Using the background equivalent radiation time (BERT) method to compare the amount of radiation received with natural background radiation received over a given period has three advantages: (1) BERT does not imply radiation risk, but rather is simply a means of comparison; (2) it emphasizes that radiation is an innate part of our environment; and (3) an answer given in terms of BERT is easy for the patient to understand.

16. Thyroid cancer continues to be the main adverse health effect of the 1986 accident at the Chernobyl nuclear power plant.

17. Three ways of indicating the amount of radiation received by a patient are (1) entrance skin exposure (ESE); (2) bone marrow dose; and (3) gonadal dose.

18. The radiation quantity, equivalent dose (EqD), enables the calculation of the effective dose (EfD).

19. Kinetic energy is energy of motion.

20. In terms of ability to penetrate biologic matter, alpha particles are less penetrating than beta particles. Because alpha particles lose energy quickly as they travel a short distance through biologic matter (e.g., into the superficial layers of the skin), they are considered virtually harmless as an external source of radiation.

Exercise 8—Essay

The questions in this exercise are intended to allow students to express their knowledge and understanding of the subject matter covered in this chapter. Because the answers may vary, determination of an answer's acceptability is left to the discretion of the instructor.

Post Test

1. Radiation protection may be defined as effective measures used by radiation workers to safeguard patients, personnel, and the general public from unnecessary exposure to ionizing radiation.

2. As low as reasonably achievable (ALARA)

3. The referring physician

4. risk

5. An effective radiation safety program

6. Electrically charged particles

7. effective

8. The sievert (Sv) is the SI unit of measure and the rem is the traditional unit of measure for the EqD and EfD.

9. B

10. D

11. The amount of radiation received by a patient

12. The electromagnetic spectrum

13. Natural sources of ionizing radiation

14. Background equivalent radiation time (BERT)

15. C

16. D

17. As an internal source of radiation

18. repeated

19. Thyroid cancer

20. Genetic damage

155

Chapter 2

Exercise 1—Crossword Puzzle

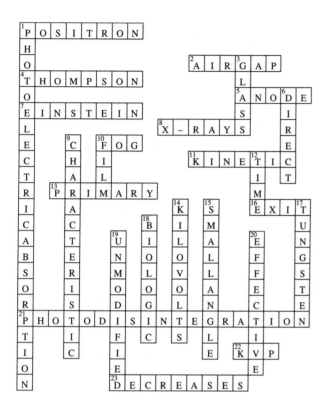

Exercise 2—Matching

1. G	6. M	11. N	16. F	21. E
2. O	7. J	12. I	17. S	22. V
3. K	8. C	13. A	18. B	23. Y
4. P	9. Q	14. R	19. T	24. X
5. D	10. L	15. H	20. U	25. W

Exercise 3—Multiple Choice

1. D	6. B	11. D	16. C	21. D
2. D	7. D	12. C	17. D	22. D
3. B	8. B	13. B	18. C	23. A
4. A	9. B	14. D	19. C	24. C
5. C	10. B	15. A	20. C	25. C

Exercise 4—True or False

1. T
2. F (direct transmission)
3. T
4. F (outer shell electron)
5. T
6. F (They must be different.)
7. T
8. F (It is not.)
9. T
10. F (increase in absorbed dose)
11. T
12. F (recoil electron)
13. T
14. T
15. F (It can cause excitation or ionization until all its kinetic energy has been spent.)
16. F (decreasing the intensity of the primary photon beam)
17. F (Characteristic radiation is also emitted from the atom.)
18. F (The minimum energy required to produce an electron-positron pair is 1.022 MeV.)
19. F (The target in the x-ray tube is also known as the *anode*.)
20. T
21. T
22. T
23. F (The Zeff of air is 7.6)
24. T
25. T

Exercise 5—Fill in the Blank

1. manmade
2. electrons, photons
3. electrical voltage
4. degrade
5. image
6. coherent (elastic, or unmodified)
7. forward, backward
8. Compton, photoelectric
9. Auger
10. absorption
11. electrons, positively
12. energy, energy
13. one third
14. intensity
15. Rayleigh, Thompson
16. darker
17. increase
18. antimatter
19. photoelectric, Compton
20. Coherent (classical, elastic, unmodified)
21. kVp
22. increases, decreases, increased
23. absorption
24. recoil
25. kinetic

Exercise 6—Labeling

A.

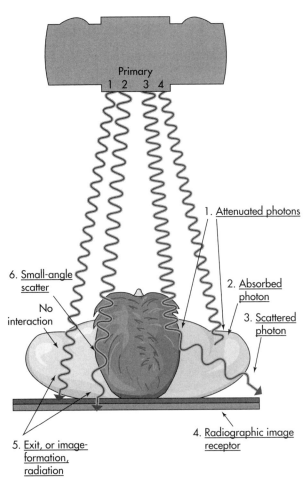

Primary − Exit = Attenuation

B.

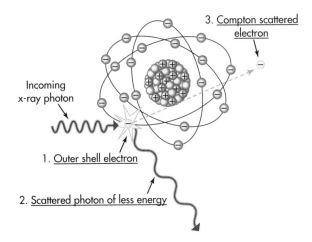

C.

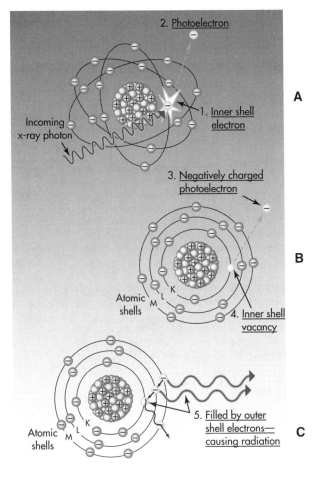

Exercise 7—Short Answer

1. Five types of interactions between x-radiation and matter are possible: (1) coherent (classical, elastic, or unmodified) scattering; (2) Compton (incoherent, inelastic, or modified) scattering; (3) photoelectric absorption; (4) pair production; and (5) photodisintegration.
2. Because the level of energy (beam quality) and the number of x-ray photons are controlled by technique factors selected by the radiographer, the radiographer is responsible for the dose the patient receives during an x-ray procedure. With a suitable understanding of these factors, radiographers can select appropriate techniques that can minimize the dose to the patient and produce a radiograph of acceptable quality.
3. The phenomenon of absorption and the differences in the absorption properties of various body structures make it possible to produce diagnostically useful radiographs in which different anatomic structures can be perceived and distinguished.
4. Reducing the amount of tissue irradiated reduces the amount of fog produced by small angle scatter. The radiographer can collimate the x-ray beam to reduce the amount of tissue irradiated.

157

5. The energy of the electrons inside a diagnostic x-ray tube is expressed in terms of the electrical voltage applied across the tube. For diagnostic radiology, this is expressed in thousands of volts, or kilovolts (kV). Moreover, because the voltage across the tube fluctuates, it usually is expressed in peak kilovoltage (kVp).

6. The minimum energy required to produce an electron-positron pair is 1.022 MeV.

7. Positive contrast media are liquid solutions that contain an element with a higher atomic number (e.g., barium or iodine) than the tissue surrounding the targeted structure or area; the media are ingested or are injected into biologic tissues or structures to be visualized.

8. Three unstable nuclei used in positron emission tomography (PET) scanning are fluorine-18 (^{18}F), carbon-11 (^{11}C), and nitrogen-13 (^{13}N).

9. A photoelectron has kinetic energy equal to the energy of the incident photon less the binding energy of the electron shell.

10. Scattered radiation can result in radiographic fog or in a biologic hazard to the radiographer.

11. The two methods most often used to limit the effects of indirectly transmitted x-ray photons are air gaps and radiographic grids.

12. During the process of coherent scattering, because the wavelengths of both incident and scattered waves are the same, no net energy is absorbed by the atom.

13. Mass density is the quantity of matter per unit volume. It generally is specified in units of kilograms per cubic meter (kg/m^3) or grams per cubic centimeter (gm/cc).

14. *Radiographic contrast* is the difference in density level between the radiographic images of objects in a radiograph.

15. Annihilation radiation is used in PET.

Chapter 3
Exercise 1—Crossword Puzzle

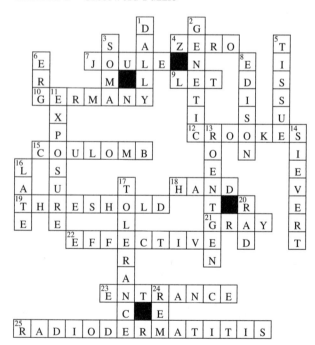

Exercise 2—Matching

1. J	6. L	11. S	16. A	21. I
2. D	7. O	12. N	17. K	22. U
3. C	8. B	13. H	18. P	23. Q
4. G	9. Y	14. T	19. F	24. R
5. E	10. M	15. W	20. X	25. V

Exercise 8—Essay
The questions in this exercise are intended to allow students to express their knowledge and understanding of the subject matter covered in this chapter. Because the answers may vary, determination of an answer's acceptability is left to the discretion of the instructor.

Post Test
1. photoelectric
2. *Attenuation* is any process that reduces the intensity of the primary photon beam directed toward a destination.
3. minimizes
4. radiographer
5. partially
6. peak kilovoltage (kVp)
7. random
8. photodisintegration
9. photoelectric absorption
10. C
11. A
12. B
13. A
14. D
15. A
16. 13.8
17. absorbed dose
18. contrast
19. all-directional
20. The term *fluorescent yield* refers to the number of characteristic x-rays emitted per inner shell vacancy.

Exercise 3—Multiple Choice

1. C	6. D	11. B	16. B	21. D
2. A	7. C	12. D	17. A	22. B
3. D	8. C	13. C	18. C	23. D
4. C	9. A	14. D	19. D	24. D
5. D	10. D	15. A	20. C	25. A

Exercise 4—True or False
1. T
2. F (The paper was coated with barium platinocyanide.)
3. T
4. T
5. F (the maximum permissible dose [MPD])
6. F (revised by the International Commission on Radiological Protection [ICRP], studies of the atomic bomb survivors)
7. T
8. F (Louis Harold Gray)
9. T
10. F (sievert and rem)
11. F (used for the radiation quantity, exposure, in air only)
12. T
13. T
14. F (number of electron-ion pairs increases)
15. T
16. F (Skin erythema dose was a crude and inaccurate means of measuring radiation exposure because the amount of radiation required to produce erythema varied from person to person.)
17. T
18. T
19. F (The higher the atomic number of a material, the more x-ray energy it absorbs.)
20. T

21. F (It may be determined and expressed in sieverts or in rems.)
22. T
23. F (The gray [Gy] or rad is used for the absorbed dose [D] measurement.)
24. T
25. T

Exercise 5—Fill in the Blank

1. W.C. (or Wilhelm Conrad) Roentgen
2. cancerous
3. erythema
4. exposure
5. organs, organ systems
6. absorbed dose
7. coulomb
8. biologic effects
9. sieverts, rem
10. risk, entire
11. radiation equivalent man
12. nonhazardous
13. different
14. quantities, units
15. workable
16. roentgen
17. 0.2, 0.1
18. roentgen
19. safe
20. SI
21. Louis Harold Gray
22. Rolf Maximilian Sievert
23. measure
24. ionization
25. temperature, pressure, humidity

Exercise 6—Labeling

A.

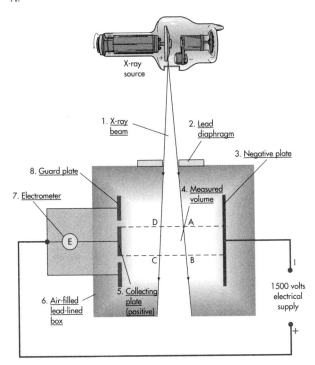

B.

Radiation Weighting Factors for Different Types and Energies of Ionizing Radiation

Radiation Type and Energy Range	Radiation Weighting Factor (W_R)
X-ray and gamma ray photons, electrons (every energy)	1. <u>1</u>
Neutrons, energy <10 keV	2. <u>5</u>
10 keV to 100 keV	3. <u>10</u>
>100 keV to 2 MeV	4. <u>20</u>
>2 MeV to 20 MeV	5. <u>10</u>
>20 MeV	6. <u>5</u>
Protons	7. <u>2</u>
Alpha particles	8. <u>20</u>

Data adapted from International Commission on Radiological Protection (ICRP): *Recommendations, ICRP publication No. 60,* New York, 1991, Pergamon Press.

C.

Summary of Radiation Quantities and Units

Type of Radiation	Quantity	SI	Traditional Unit	Measuring Medium	Radiation Effect Measured
X-radiation or gamma	1. Exposure (X)	Coulomb per kilogram (C/kg)	Roentgen (R)	Air	Ionization of air radiation
All ionizing radiations	2. Absorbed dose (D)	Gray (Gy)	Rad	Any object	Amount of energy per unit mass absorbed by object
All ionizing radiations	3. Equivalent dose (EqD)	Sievert (Sv)	Rem	Body tissue	Biologic effects
All ionizing radiations	4. Effective dose (Efd)	Sievert (Sv)	Rem	Body tissue	Biologic effects

Exercise 7—Short Answer

1. Thomas A. Edison discontinued his x-ray research because of the severe injuries and death of his friend, Clarence Dally, which were attributed to radiation-induced cancer.
2. Skin erythema dose was the unit used for measuring radiation exposure from 1900 to 1930.
3. Short-term (early or acute) somatic effects of ionizing radiation are effects that appear within minutes, hours, days, or weeks of radiation exposure. Long-term, or late, somatic effects appear months or years after exposure to ionizing radiation.
4. Tolerance dose is a radiation dose to which occupationally exposed persons could be continuously subjected without any apparent harmful acute effects, such as erythema of the skin.
5. Maximum permissible dose (or MPD) replaced tolerance dose for radiation protection purposes in the 1950s.
6. In the late 1970s, dose limits were calculated and established to ensure that the risk from radiation exposure acquired while on the job did not exceed risks encountered in "safe" occupations, such as clerical work (i.e., approximately 10^{-4} per year).
7. The Bragg-Gray theory relates the ionization produced in a small cavity within an irradiated medium or object to the energy absorbed in that medium as a result of its radiation exposure. Thus with the use of appropriate correction factors, the theory essentially links the determination of the absorbed radiation dose in a medium to a relatively simple measurement of ionization charge. The Bragg-Gray theory is the most important theory in radiation dosimetry.
8. When the human body is exposed to ionizing radiation, absorbed energy is responsible for any biologic damage to the tissues resulting from this exposure.
9. For precise measurement of radiation exposure in radiography, the total amount of ionization an x-ray beam produces in a known mass of air must be obtained. This type of direct measurement is accomplished in an accredited calibration laboratory using a standard or free air ionization chamber.
10. The radiation weighting factors are selected by national and international scientific advisory bodies (NCRP, ICRP) and are based on quality factors and linear energy transfer.
11. If the absorbed dose is stated in rads, the equivalent number of gray may be determined by dividing the rad value by 100.
12. If the absorbed dose is stated in gray, the number of rads may be determined by multiplying the gray value by 100.
13. Coulomb per kilogram (C/kg) or roentgen (R) is used for calibration of x-ray equipment because x-ray output is measured directly with an ionization chamber.
14. If the radiation exposure is given in R, it can be converted to C/kg by multiplying by 2.58×10^{-4}.
15. If the radiation exposure is given in C/kg, it can be converted to R by dividing by 2.58×10^{-4}.

Exercise 8—Essay

The questions in this exercise are intended to allow students to express their knowledge and understanding of the subject matter covered in this chapter. Because the answers may vary, determination of an answer's acceptability is left to the discretion of the instructor.

Exercise 9—Calculation Problems

A.

1. 8000 rads = 8000 ÷ 100 rads per Gy = 80 Gy
2. 8 rads = 8 ÷ 100 rads per Gy = 0.08 Gy
3. 450 rads = 450 ÷ 100 rads per Gy = 4.5 Gy
4. 4.5 rads = 4.5 ÷ 100 rads per Gy = 0.045 Gy
5. 375 rads = 375 ÷ 100 rads per Gy = 3.75 Gy
6. 7 Gy = 7 × 100 rads per Gy = 700 rads
7. 25 Gy = 25 × 100 rads per Gy = 2500 rads
8. 0.4 Gy = 0.4 × 100 rads per Gy = 40 rads
9. 0.087 Gy = 0.087 × 100 rads per Gy = 8.7 rads
10. 0.96 Gy = 0.96 × 100 rads per Gy = 96 rads

B.

1.

Radiation Type	D	×	W$_R$	=	EqD
X-radiation	0.6 Gy	×	1	=	0.6 Sv
Fast neutrons	0.25 Gy	×	20	=	5 Sv
Alpha particles	0.4 Gy	×	20	=	8 Sv
				Total EqD = 13.6 Sv	

2.

Radiation Type	D	×	W$_R$	=	EqD
X-radiation	0.3 Gy	×	1	=	0.3 Sv
Fast neutrons	0.28 Gy	×	20	=	5.6 Sv
Gamma rays	0.8 Gy	×	1	=	0.8 Sv
Protons	0.9 Gy	×	2	=	1.8 Sv
Alpha particles	0.4 Gy	×	20	=	8 Sv
				Total EqD = 16.5 Sv	

3.

Radiation Type	D	×	W$_R$	=	EqD
X-radiation	7 rads	×	1	=	7 rem
Fast neutrons	2 rads	×	20	=	40 rem
Alpha particles	5 rads	×	20	=	100 rem
				Total EqD = 147 rem	

4.

Radiation Type	D	×	W$_R$	=	EqD
X-radiation	3 rads	×	1	=	3 rem
Fast neutrons	0.35 rads	×	20	=	7 rem
Gamma rays	6 rads	×	1	=	6 rem
Protons	2.5 rads	×	2	=	5 rem
Alpha particles	8 rads	×	20	=	160 rem
				Total EqD = 181 rem	

5.

Radiation Type	D	×	W$_R$	=	EqD
X-radiation	0.6 Gy	×	1	=	0.6 Sv
Fast neutrons, energy <10 keV	0.2 Gy	×	5	=	1 Sv
Gamma rays	4 Gy	×	1	=	4 Sv
Protons	0.8 Gy	×	2	=	1.6 Sv
Alpha particles	6 Gy	×	20	=	120 Sv
				Total EqD = 127.2 Sv	

C.

	D	×	W$_R$	×	W$_T$	= EfD
1.	0.5 Gy	×	20	×	0.05	= 0.5 Sv
2.	0.4 Gy	×	1	×	0.2	= 0.08 Sv
3.	6 rads	×	20	×	0.12	= 14.4 rem
4.	25 rads	×	1	×	0.05	= 1.25 rem
5.	0.9 Gy	×	1	×	0.12	= 0.108 Sv

D.

	Number Exposed	×	Average EfD (Sv)	=	ColEfD
1.	400	×	0.2	=	80 person-sievert (80 × 100 = 8000 man-rem)
2.	300	×	0.17	=	51 person-sievert (51 × 100 = 5100 man-rem)
3.	250	×	0.24	=	60 person-sievert (60 × 100 = 6000 man-rem)
4.	1000	×	0.1	=	100 person-sievert (100 × 100 = 10,000 man-rem)
5.	100	×	0.3	=	30 person-sievert (30 × 100 = 3000 man-rem)

Post Test

1. Number exposed × Average EfD = ColEfD
   $400 \times 0.2\,\text{Sv} = 80$ person-sievert $(80 \times 100 = 8000$ man-rem)
2. Effective dose (EfD)
3. Linear energy transfer (LET)
4. The radiation quantity, exposure (X), is expressed in coulombs per kilogram (C/kg) in the SI system and in roentgen (R) in the traditional system.
5. Leukemia
6. Wilhelm Conrad Roentgen
7.

Radiation Type	D	×	W$_R$	=	EqD
X-radiation	5 Gy	×	1	=	5 Sv
Fast neutrons	0.3 Gy	×	20	=	1.5 Sv
Alpha particles	0.7 Gy	×	20	=	14 Sv
				Total EqD =	20.5 Sv

8. $D \times W_R \times W_T = \text{EfD}$
   $5\,\text{Gy} \times 1 \times 0.12 = 0.6\,\text{Sv}$
9. 800
10. $\text{EqD} = D \times W_R$
11. A
12. C
13. Skin erythema
14. coulomb (c)
15. D
16. 10
17. centigray (cGy)
18. cancerous
19. Radiation exposure received by workers in the course of their professional responsibilities
20. The energy deposited in biologic tissue by ionizing radiation

Chapter 4

Exercise 1—Crossword Puzzle

Exercise 2—Matching

1. D	6. C	11. E	16. J	21. Y
2. M	7. N	12. R	17. U	22. X
3. L	8. A	13. H	18. I	23. V
4. K	9. P	14. T	19. B	24. S
5. F	10. G	15. O	20. W	25. Q

Exercise 3—Multiple Choice

1. C	6. B	11. A	16. B	21. D
2. B	7. D	12. C	17. A	22. C
3. C	8. B	13. B	18. D	23. B
4. B	9. C	14. B	19. D	24. B
5. D	10. B	15. C	20. C	25. C

Exercise 4—True or False

1. T
2. F (80% to 85%)
3. T
4. F (The body's primary defense mechanism against infection and disease are antibodies.)
5. T
6. F (hydrogen bonds)
7. T
8. T
9. F (occur in the cytoplasm)
10. T
11. T
12. T
13. F (It is frail and semipermeable.)
14. T
15. T
16. T
17. F (during metaphase)
18. T
19. T
20. F (Glucose is the primary energy source.)
21. T
22. F (Cells are essential for life.)
23. T
24. F (Proteins contain the most carbon.)
25. F (Carbohydrates are most abundant in the liver and in muscle tissue.)

Exercise 5—Fill in the Blank

1. cell
2. homeostasis
3. 24
4. amino acids
5. repair enzymes
6. Hormones
7. liver, muscle
8. DNA
9. osmotic
10. fraternal
11. DNA
12. high
13. fluid
14. metabolism
15. metabolism

16. Ribosomes
17. catalytic, repair
18. macromolecules
19. nucleus
20. endoplasmic reticulum

21. replication
22. Lysosomes
23. Oxidative
24. Salts
25. electrolytes

Exercise 6—Labeling
A.

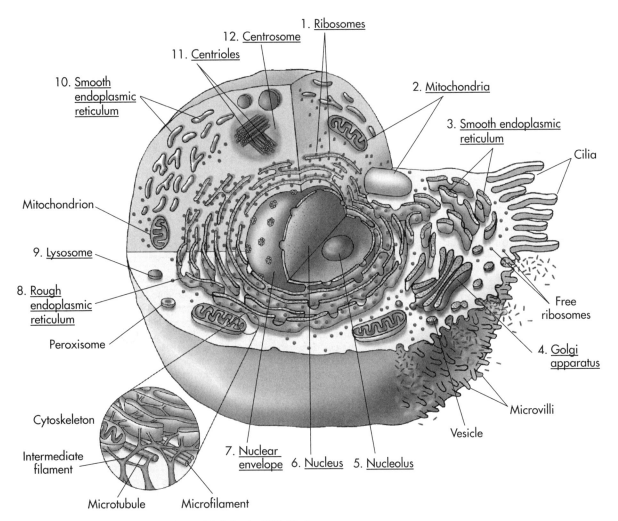

1. Ribosomes
12. Centrosome
11. Centrioles
10. Smooth endoplasmic reticulum
2. Mitochondria
3. Smooth endoplasmic reticulum
Cilia
Mitochondrion
9. Lysosome
8. Rough endoplasmic reticulum
Peroxisome
Free ribosomes
4. Golgi apparatus
Microvilli
Vesicle
Cytoskeleton
Intermediate filament
7. Nuclear envelope
6. Nucleus
5. Nucleolus
Microtubule
Microfilament

From Thibodeau A: *Anatomy and physiology,* ed 5, St Louis, 2003, Mosby.

B.

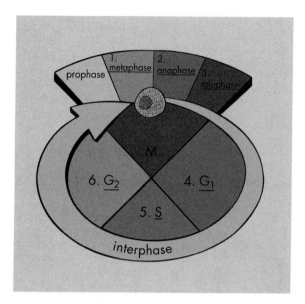

From Bushong SC: *Radiologic science for technologists: physics, biology, and protection,* ed 8, St. Louis, 2004, Elsevier.

C.

Summary of Cell Components

Title	Site	Activity
1. Cell membrane	Cytoplasm	Functions as a barricade to protect cellular contents from their environment and controls the passage of water and other materials into and out of the cell; performs many additional functions such as elimination of wastes and refining of material for energy through breakdown of the materials
2. Endoplasmic reticulum	Cytoplasm	Enables the cell to communicate with the extracellular environment and transfers food from one part of the cell to another
3. Golgi apparatus	Cytoplasm	Unites large carbohydrate molecules and combines them with proteins to form glycoproteins and transports enzymes and hormones through the cell membrane so that they can exit the cell, enter the bloodstream, and be carried to areas of the body in which they are required
4. Mitochondria	Cytoplasm	Produce energy for cellular activity by breaking down nutrients through a process of oxidation
5. Lysosomes	Cytoplasm	Dispose of large particles such as bacteria and food as well as smaller particles; also contain hydrolytic enzymes that can break down and digest proteins, certain carbohydrates, and the cell itself if the lysosome's surrounding membrane breaks
6. Ribosomes	Cytoplasm	Manufacture the various proteins that cells require
7. Centrosomes	Cytoplasm	Believed to play some part in the formation of the mitotic spindle during cell division
8. DNA	Nucleus	Contains the genetic material, controls cell division and multiplication and also biochemical reactions that occur within the living cell
9. Nucleolus	Nucleus	Holds a large amount of RNA

Exercise 7—Short Answer

1. To ensure efficient cell operation, the body must provide food as a source of raw material for the release of energy, supply oxygen to help break down the food, and have enough water to transport inorganic substances such as calcium and sodium into and out of the cell.

2. Metabolism involves chemical reactions in the body that modify food for cellular use.

3. Proteins are formed by combining amino acids into long, chainlike molecular complexes. In these complexes a chemical link, called *a peptide bond,* connects each amino acid. Protein production, or *protein synthesis,* involves 22 different amino acids. The order of arrangement of these amino acids determines the precise function of each protein molecule.

4. Enzymatic proteins function as *organic catalysts,* agents that affect the speed of chemical reactions without being altered themselves. Enzymatic proteins control the cell's various physiologic activities. Enzymes cause an increase in cellular activity, which in turn speeds up biochemical reactions to meet the needs of the cell. Therefore proper cell functioning depends on enzymes.

5. Lipids are fats or fatlike substances that are present in all body tissue. They perform many functions; for example, they (1) act as reservoirs for long-term storage of energy; (2) insulate and guard the body against the environment; (3) support and protect organs such as the eyes and kidneys; (4) provide essential substances for growth and development; (5) lubricate the joints; and (6) assist in the digestive process.

6. Ribosomes function as protein factories for the cell; they manufacture (synthesize) the various proteins that cells require using the blueprints provided by messenger ribonucleic acid (mRNA).

7. Inside the cell, water is indispensable for metabolic activity because it is the medium in which the chemical reactions that are the bases of these activities occur. It also acts as a solvent, keeping compounds dissolved so that they can more easily interact and their concentration can be regulated. Outside the cell, water functions as a transport vehicle for minerals the cell uses or eliminates. In addition, water maintains a constant body core temperature of 37° C and lubricates both the digestive system and the skeletal articulations (joints). Organs such as the brain and lungs are also protected by a cushion of water.

8. The nucleus controls cell division and multiplication and the biochemical reactions that occur inside the cell. By directing protein synthesis, the nucleus plays an essential role in active transport, metabolism, growth and heredity.

9. Four distinct phases of the cellular life cycle are identifiable: M (mitosis phase), G_1 (pre-DNA synthesis phase), S (synthesis phase), and G_2 (post-DNA synthesis phase).

10. Carbohydrates are referred to as *saccharides.* A monosaccharide is a simple sugar molecule (e.g., glucose). A *disaccharide* is made up of two units of a simple sugar linked together (e.g., sucrose [cane sugar]). A *polysaccharide* is composed of several or many molecules of a simple sugar.

11. The four major classes of organic compounds in the human body are proteins, carbohydrates, lipids (fats), and nucleic acids.

12. Deoxyribonucleic acid (DNA) is a type of nucleic acid that carries the genetic information necessary for cell replication and directs the building of proteins.

13. Structural proteins, such as those found in muscle, provide the body with its shape and form and are a source of heat and energy.

14. The nucleus of a cell controls cell division and multiplication and the biochemical reactions that occur within the cell. By directing protein synthesis, the nucleus plays an essential role in active transport, metabolism, growth, and heredity.

15. Hormones are chemical secretions manufactured by various endocrine glands and carried by the bloodstream to influence the activities of other parts of the body. Hormones produced by the thyroid gland control metabolism throughout the body.

Exercise 8—Essay

The questions in this exercise are intended to allow students to express their knowledge and understanding of the subject matter covered in this chapter. Because the answers may vary, determination of an answer's acceptability is left to the discretion of the instructor.

Post Test

1. matter
2. organic
3. repair enzymes
4. nitrogenous
5. water
6. The DNA macromolecule is composed of two long sugar-phosphate chains that twist around each other in a double-helix configuration; these chains are linked by pairs of nitrogenous organic bases at the sugar molecules of the chain, forming a tightly coiled structure resembling a twisted ladder or spiral staircase. The sugar-phosphate compounds are the side rails and the pairs of nitrogenous bases, which consist of complementary chemicals, are the steps, or rungs, of the DNA ladderlike structure. Hydrogen bonds attach the bases to each other, joining the two side rails of the DNA ladder.
7. mapping
8. C
9. C
10. During metaphase
11. Ribosomes synthesize the various proteins that cells require.
12. Approximately 30,000
13. The affected cells will function abnormally or die.
14. 22
15. a nucleotide
16. DNA
17. cytoplasm
18. Interphase
19. Lipids
20. The cell membrane surrounds the cell, functions as a barricade, and controls the passage of water and other materials into and out of the cell.

Chapter 5

Exercise 1—Crossword Puzzle

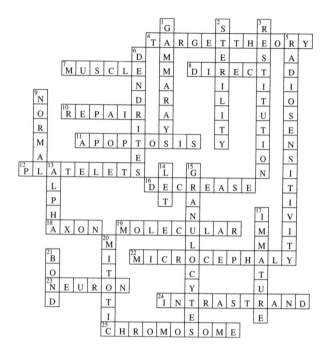

Exercise 2—Matching

1. N	6. L	11. B	16. Y	21. S
2. O	7. A	12. G	17. P	22. Q
3. H	8. K	13. M	18. W	23. X
4. D	9. I	14. J	19. R	24. U
5. E	10. F	15. C	20. V	25. T

Exercise 3—Multiple Choice

1. B	6. D	11. C	16. B
2. B	7. D	12. A	17. C
3. A	8. C	13. A	18. A
4. D	9. D	14. A	19. A
5. A	10. A	15. B	20. C

Exercise 4—True or False

1. F (can be damaged by radiation)
2. T
3. F (vary among the different types of ionizing radiation)
4. T
5. F (high-LET radiation)

6. F (are basically unstable)
7. T
8. F (contains large numbers if immature, unspecialized cells, and is therefore radiosensitive)
9. T
10. T
11. F (deoxyribonucleic acid [DNA])
12. T
13. F (can adversely affect cell division)
14. T
15. T
16. T
17. F (The presence of free radicals dramatically increases the amount of biologic damage produced.)
18. F (X-ray photons may interact with and ionize water molecules in the human body.)
19. T
20. T
21. F (different types of cells and tissues, which vary in their degree of radiosensitivity)
22. F (In radiotherapy the presence of oxygen plays a significant role in radiosensitivity.)
23. F (the less sensitive it is to radiation)
24. T
25. T

Exercise 5—Fill in the Blank

1. cellular
2. energy
3. sublethal
4. mass, charge
5. internal
6. permanent
7. hydroxyl
8. Gene
9. Radiosensitivity
10. ionizing radiation
11. infection
12. platelets
13. Granulocytes
14. decrease
15. mitosis
16. radiosensitive
17. radiosensitive
18. microcephaly (small head circumference), mental retardation
19. insensitive
20. radiosensitive
21. dies, restored
22. 2 (200)
23. 5 to 6 (500 to 600)
24. immature, susceptible
25. 0.25 (25)

Exercise 6—Labeling

A.

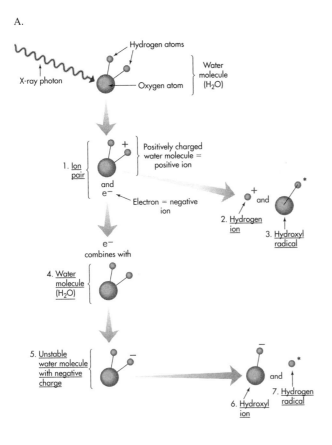

B.

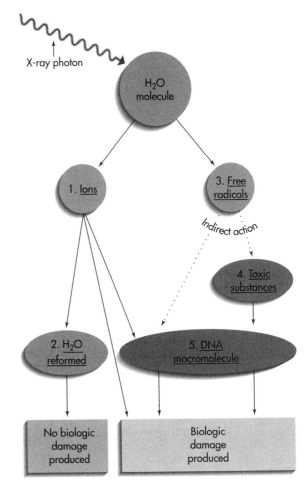

C.

Examples of Radiosensitive and Radioinsensitive Cells

Radiosensitive Cells	Radioinsensitive Cells
1. <u>Basal cells of the skin</u>	4. <u>Brain cells</u>
2. <u>Intestinal crypt cells</u>	5. <u>Muscle cells</u>
3. <u>Reproductive (germ) cells</u>	6. <u>Nerve cells</u>

Exercise 7—Short Answer

1. High-energy charged particles (e.g., alpha and beta particles and protons) ionize by interacting electromagnetically with orbital electrons. For example, an alpha particle that carries an electrical charge of plus two strongly attracts the negatively charged electron as it passes by.

2. Characteristics that vary (e.g., charge, mass, and energy) among the different types of radiations determine the extent to which different radiation modalities transfer energy into biologic tissue.

3. LET generally is expressed in units of kiloelectron volts (keV) per micron (1 micron [μm] = 10^{-6} m).

4. Repair enzymes usually can reverse the cellular damage caused by low-LET radiation because low-LET radiation generally causes sublethal damage to DNA.

5. A free radical is a solitary atom or, most often, a combination of atoms that behaves as an extremely reactive single entity because it has an unpaired electron.

6. All cells in the body other than female and male germ cells are classified as somatic cells.

7. Oxygen enhances the effects of ionizing radiation on biologic tissue by increasing tissue radiosensitivity. If oxygen is present when a tissue is irradiated, more free radicals are formed in the tissue; this increases the potential for indirect damage from radiation.

8. Damage to the cell's nucleus from ionizing radiation reveals itself in one of the following ways: instant death; reproductive death; apoptosis, or programmed cell death (interphase death); mitotic, or genetic, death; mitotic delay; interference of function; and chromosome breakage.

9. With *direct action*, biologic damage occurs as a result of ionization of atoms on master, or key, molecules (DNA), which can cause these molecules to become inactive or functionally altered. *Indirect action* refers to the effects produced by reactive free radicals created by the interaction of radiation with water (H_2O) molecules. These unstable, highly reactive agents have the potential to substantially disrupt master molecules, resulting in cell death.

10. If the nucleus in an adult nerve cell is destroyed by exposure to ionizing radiation, the cell dies and is never restored.

11. Even small doses of ionizing radiation (e.g., as low as 0.1 Gy [10 rads]) may cause menstrual irregularities, such as delay or suppression of menstruation.

12. Ionizing radiation interacts randomly with matter. Consequently, exposure to radiation produces a variety of structural changes in biologic tissue. Seven of these possible changes are: (1) a single-strand break in one chromosome; (2) a single-strand break in one chromatid; (3) a single-strand break in separate chromosomes; (4) a strand break in separate chromatids; (5) more than one break in the same chromosome; (6) more than one break in the same chromatid; and (7) chromosome stickiness, or clumping.

13. Radiation damage is observed on three levels: molecular, cellular, and organic.

14. Ionizing radiation causes complete chromosome breakage when two direct hits occur in the same rung of the DNA macromolecule.

15. In 1906 two French scientists, J. Bergonié and L. Tribondeau, observed the effects of ionizing radiation on the testicular germ cells of rabbits they had exposed to x-rays. They established that radiosensitivity was a function of the metabolic state of the cell receiving the exposure. Their findings eventually became known as the Bergonié-Tribondeau Law, which states that the radiosensitivity of cells is directly proportional to their reproductive activity and inversely proportional to their degree of differentiation.

Exercise 8—Essay

The questions in this exercise are intended to allow students to express their knowledge and understanding of the subject matter covered in this chapter. Because the answers may vary, determination of an answer's acceptability is left to the discretion of the instructor.

Post Test

1. The following formula is used:

    Dose in Gy from 250 kVp

    x-rays (reference radiation)

    = Relative biologic effectiveness (RBE)

    Dose in Gy of test radiation

    $21 \div 7 = 3$

    RBE = 3

2. Water

3. apoptosis

4. LET is the amount of energy transferred on average by incident radiation to an object per unit length of track through the object. It is expressed in units of keV/μm.

5. Oxygen enhancement ratio (OER)

6. direct

7. C

8. D

9. target

10. indirect

11. lymphocytes

12. Bergonié-Tribondeau Law

13. mutations

14. A cell survival curve is used to display the radiosensitivity of a particular type of cell, which helps determine the types of cancer cells that will respond to radiation therapy.

15. bond

16. a measurable hematologic depression

17. repopulate

18. blood count

19. mental retardation

20. Ionizing radiation causes complete chromosome breakage when two direct hits occur in the same rung of the DNA macromolecule.

Chapter 6

Exercise 1—Crossword Puzzle

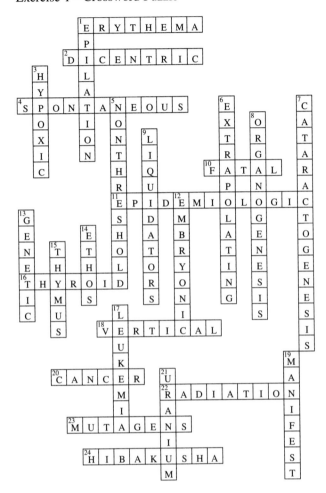

Exercise 2—Matching

1. O	6. N	11. Y	16. F	21. U
2. E	7. D	12. H	17. Q	22. W
3. M	8. G	13. X	18. C	23. S
4. K	9. J	14. B	19. V	24. R
5. A	10. I	15. P	20. L	25. T

Exercise 3—Multiple Choice

1. A	6. D	11. A	16. D	21. D
2. B	7. D	12. C	17. A	22. D
3. B	8. D	13. A	18. D	23. A
4. C	9. D	14. D	19. B	24. B
5. B	10. C	15. A	20. A	25. C

Exercise 4—True or False

1. T
2. F (nonthreshold relationship)
3. F (nonthreshold)
4. T
5. T
6. F (decrease)
7. F (3 to 4 Gy [300 to 400 rads])
8. T
9. T
10. F (carcinogenesis)
11. F (Large dose of densely ionizing, high-LET radiation is delivered to a large or radiosensitive area of the body.)
12. F (high-LET radiation exposure)
13. T
14. F (No conclusive proof exists.)
15. T
16. F (Whole-body equivalent doses greater than 12 Gy [1200 rads] are considered fatal.)
17. T
18. T
19. F (Survivors have demonstrated late deterministic and stochastic effects of ionizing radiation.)
20. T
21. T
22. F (Repeated radiation injury does have a cumulative effect.)
23. F (Cancer is the most important late somatic effect caused by exposure to ionizing radiation.)
24. T
25. T

Exercise 5—Fill in the Blank

1. somatic, genetic
2. linear, threshold
3. overestimate, underestimate
4. early, late somatic
5. hematopoietic, gastrointestinal, cerebrovascular
6. nausea, vomiting
7. death
8. controversial
9. cancer
10. breast
11. 1.56, (156)
12. calcium
13. malignancy
14. mutagens
15. 4:1, 10:1
16. leukemia
17. cancer-causing
18. follow-up studies
19. thyroid, iodine
20. reconstructing
21. cancer
22. lens
23. radiosensitive, damaged
24. first, stem
25. death

Exercise 6—Labeling

A.

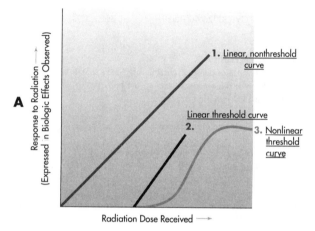

B.

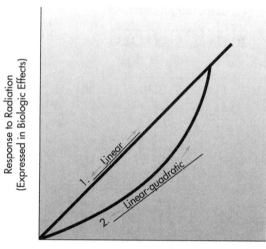

1. Linear, nonthreshold curve

Linear threshold curve

2.

3. Nonlinear threshold curve

1. Linear

2. Linear-quadratic

Radiation Dose

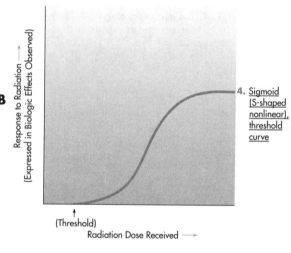

4. Sigmoid (S-shaped nonlinear), threshold curve

(Threshold)

C.

Overview of Acute Radiation Lethality

Stage	Dose Gy (Rads)	Average Survival Time	Symptoms
1. Prodromal	1 (100)	—	Nausea, vomiting, diarrhea, fatigue, leukopenia
2. Latent	1–100 (100–10,000)	—	None
3. Hematopoietic	1–10 (100–1000)	6 to 8 wk (doses over 2 Gy)	Nausea; vomiting; diarrhea; decrease in number of red blood cells, white blood cells, and platelets in the circulating blood; hemorrhage; infection
4. Gastrointestinal	6–10 (600–1000)	3–10 days	Severe nausea, vomiting, diarrhea, fever, fatigue, loss of appetite, lethargy, anemia, leukopenia, hemorrhage, infection, electrolytic imbalance, and emaciation
5. Cerebrovascular	5 and above (5000 and above)	Several hours to 2 or 3 days	Same as hematopoietic and gastrointestinal, excessive nervousness, confusion, lack of coordination, loss of vision, a burning sensation of the skin, loss of consciousness, disorientation, shock, periods of agitation alternating with stupor, edema, loss of equilibrium, meningitis, prostration, respiratory distress, vasculitis, coma

Exercise 7—Short Answer

1. With regard to ionizing radiation, if a threshold relationship exists between the radiation dose and a biologic response, no biologic effects are observed below a certain radiation dose, or level. Biologic effects are observed only when the threshold level, or dose, is reached. A nonthreshold relationship means that any radiation dose will produce a biologic effect. No radiation dose is believed to be absolutely safe.

2. Laboratory experiments on animals and data from human populations observed after acute high doses of radiation provide the foundation for a linear, threshold curve of radiation-dose response.

3. ARS presents in four major response stages: prodromal or initial stage, latent period, manifest illness, and recovery or death.

4. The three forms of ARS are hematopoietic syndrome (bone marrow syndrome), gastrointestinal syndrome, and cerebrovascular syndrome.

5. Using all data available on high radiation exposure, members of the scientific and medical communities have determined that three categories of health effects require study at low-level exposures: cancer induction, damage to the unborn from irradiation in utero, and genetic effects.

6. Three types of late somatic effects are carcinogenesis, cataractogenesis, and embryologic effects (birth defects).

7. Evidence for human radiation cataractogenesis comes from observation of small groups of people who accidentally received substantial doses to the eyes. These groups include Japanese atomic bomb survivors, nuclear physicists working with cyclotrons between 1932 and 1960, and patients undergoing radiotherapy who received significant high exposures to the eyes during treatment.

8. Fetal radiosensitivity declines as gestation in human beings progresses. The developing fetus is less sensitive to ionizing radiation exposure during the second and third trimesters of pregnancy than in the first trimester. However, congenital abnormalities and functional disorders (e.g., sterility) may be caused by radiation exposure. Leukemia may be induced by exposure to radiation during the second and third trimesters.

9. Mutagens, such as ionizing radiation, can increase the incidence of mutations that occur as part of the natural order of events.

10. Researchers commonly use two models for extrapolation of risk from high-dose to low-dose data. These are the linear and linear-quadratic models.

11. The only concrete evidence that ionizing radiation causes genetic effects comes from extensive experiments with fruit flies and mice at high radiation doses.

12. Point mutations (genetic mutations at the molecular level) may be either dominant (probably expressed in the offspring) or recessive (probably not expressed for several generations). Radiation is thought to cause primarily recessive mutations, if any.

13. To minimize the possibility of genetic effects in medical imaging professionals and patients, gonadal shielding must be used effectively, and all radiation exposure must be kept as low as reasonably achievable (ALARA).

14. Gestation in human beings is divided into three stages: preimplantation, which corresponds to 0 to 9 days; organogenesis, which corresponds to 10 days to 6 weeks after conception; and the fetal stage, which corresponds from 6 weeks to term.

15. Most lethal dose (LD) data represent an estimate of the role played by radiation in fatalities that involved other factors. Specifications of lethal effects are further complicated by the medical treatment the patient may receive during the prodromal and latent stages, before many of the symptoms of ARS appear. When medical treatment is given promptly, the patient is supported through initial symptoms, but the question of long-term survival may be delayed. Therefore survival over a 60-day period may be a more relevant indicator of outcome for human beings than survival over a 30-day period. This is the reason LD 50/60 may be more accurate for human beings.

Exercise 8—Essay

The questions in this exercise are intended to allow students to express their knowledge and understanding of the subject matter covered in this chapter. Because the answers may vary, determination of an answer's acceptability is left to the discretion of the instructor.

Post Test

1. organogenesis
2. cancer
3. during the embryonic stage of development
4. 8
5. absolute risk model
6. manifest illness
7. linear, nonthreshold curve
8. C
9. D
10. Nonstochastic (deterministic) somatic effects are biologic somatic effects of ionizing radiation that can be directly related to the dose received. These cell-killing effects exhibit a threshold dose below which the effect does not normally occur and above which the severity of the biologic damage increases as the dose increases.
11. The sigmoid, or S-shaped (nonlinear), threshold curve of the radiation dose-response relationship is generally used in radiation therapy to demonstrate high-dose cellular response.
12. Without effective physical monitoring devices, biologic criteria such as the occurrence of nausea and vomiting played an important role in the identification of radiation casualties in the first 2 days after the accident at the Chernobyl nuclear power plant.
13. gastrointestinal
14. 3 to 4 Gy (300 to 400 rads)
15. Ionizing radiation can induce genetic damage by altering the essential base coding sequence of DNA.
16. Repeated radiation injury has a cumulative effect.
17. greatest
18. With reference to ionizing radiation, the term *threshold* means that no biologic effects are observed below a certain radiation level, or dose. Biologic effects are observed only when the threshold level, or dose, is reached.
19. 50, (500)
20. Thyroid cancer is considered the most pronounced health consequence of the accident at the Chernobyl nuclear power plant.

Chapter 7

Exercise 1—Crossword Puzzle

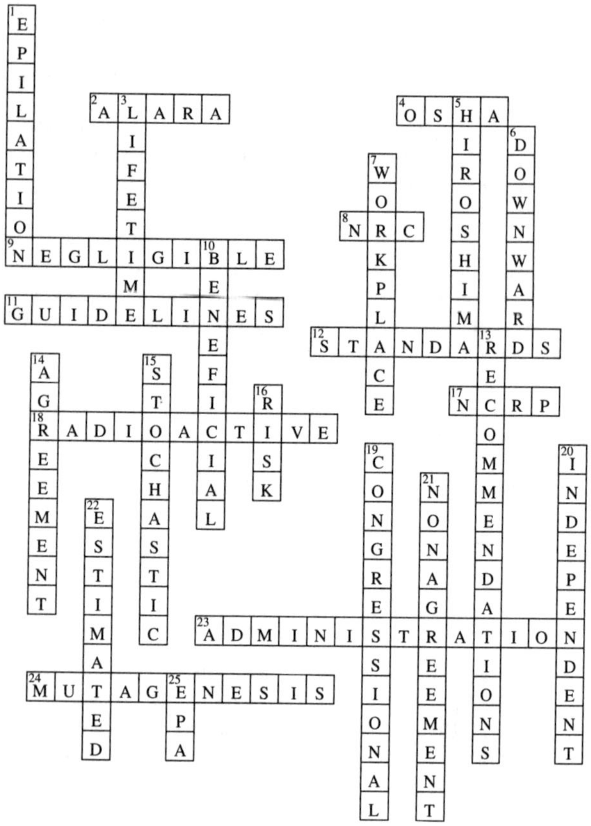

1 EPILATION
2 ALARA
3 LIFETIME
4 OSHA
5 HIROSHIMA
6 DOWNWARD
7 WORKPLACE
8 NRC
9 NEGLIGIBLE
10 BENEFICIAL
11 GUIDELINES
12 STANDARDS
13 RECOMMENDATIONS
14 AGREEMENT
15 STOCHASTIC
16 RISK
17 NCRP
18 RADIOACTIVE
19 CONGRESSIONAL
20 INDEPENDENT
21 NONAGREEMENT
22 ESTIMATED
23 ADMINISTRATION
24 MUTAGENESIS
25 EPA

Exercise 2—Matching

1. X	6. J	11. C	16. U	21. Y
2. N	7. Q	12. S	17. O	22. F
3. T	8. P	13. M	18. V	23. A
4. G	9. B	14. D	19. E	24. L
5. R	10. I	15. K	20. H	25. W

Exercise 3—Multiple Choice

1. B	6. D	11. C	16. A	21. A
2. D	7. A	12. B	17. C	22. D
3. B	8. A	13. A	18. B	23. D
4. D	9. D	14. C	19. D	24. B
5. A	10. A	15. B	20. D	25. B

Exercise 4—True or False

1. F (It does not.)
2. T
3. T
4. F (It does not.)
5. T
6. F (Do need to have an effective radiation safety program)
7. T
8. T
9. F (It is not; it conducts an ongoing electronic products radiation control program.)
10. T
11. T
12. T
13. F (It does not, the Environmental Protection Agency [EPA] does.)
14. T
15. T
16. T
17. F (The embryo-fetus is particularly sensitive.)
18. F (Effective dose limits do not include background radiation or exposure acquired when a worker undergoing medical imaging procedures.)
19. T
20. F (an active participant)
21. T
22. F (The Right-to-Know Act requires employers to evaluate their workplace for hazardous agents and provide training and written information to their employees.)
23. T
24. T
25. T

Exercise 5—Fill in the Blank

1. previous, existing, new
2. dose limits
3. nongovernmental, nonprofit
4. biologic, risk
5. radon
6. radioactive
7. Radiation Safety
8. dose limits
9. optimization
10. stochastic
11. 1, (0.1)
12. risk
13. random
14. mutations
15. linear, linear quadratic
16. risk
17. greater
18. 0.4, (40)
19. 8, 15
20. cancer, genetic
21. whole body
22. nonoccupationally
23. same
24. external, internal
25. 50, (5), 10

Exercise 6—Labeling

A.

Summary of Radiation Protection Standards Organizations

Organization	Function
1. ICRP	Evaluates information on biologic effects of radiation and provides radiation protection guidance through general recommendations on occupational and public dose limits
2. NCRP	Reviews regulations formulated by the ICRP and decides ways to include those recommendations into U.S. radiation protection criteria
3. UNSCEAR	Evaluates human and environmental ionizing radiation exposure and derives radiation risk assessments from epidemiologic data and research conclusions; provides information to organizations such as the ICRP for evaluation
4. NAS/NRC-BEIR	Reviews studies of biologic effects of ionizing radiation and risk assessment and provides the information to organizations such as the ICRP for evaluation

B.

Summary of U.S. Regulatory Agencies

Agency	Function
1. NRC	Oversees the nuclear energy industry, enforces radiation protection standards, publishes its rules and regulations in Title 10 of the U.S. Code of Federal Regulations, enters into written agreements with state governments permitting the state to license and regulate the use of radioisotopes and certain other material within that state
2. Agreement states	Enforces radiation protection regulations through their respective health departments
3. EPA	Facilitates the development and enforcement of regulations pertaining to the control of radiation in the environment
4. FDA	Conducts an ongoing product radiation control program, regulating the design and manufacture of electronic products, including x-ray equipment
5. OSHA	Functions as a monitoring agency in places of employment, predominantly in industry

C.

Summary of the National Council on Radiation Protection and Measurements (NCRP) Recommendations*†
(NCRP Report No. 116)

A. Occupational exposures‡		
1. Effective dose limits		
a. Annual	1. 50 mSv	(5 rem)
b. Cumulative	2. 10 mSv × age	1 rem × age
2. Equivalent dose annual limits for tissues and organs		
a. Lens of eye	3. 150 mSv	(15 rem)
b. Localized areas of the skin, hands, and feet	4. 500 mSv	(50 rem)
B. Guidance for emergency occupational exposure‡ (see Section 14, NCRP #116)		
C. Public exposures (annual)		
1. Effective dose limit, continuous or frequent exposure‡	5. 1 mSv	(0.1 rem)
2. Effective dose limit, infrequent exposure‡	6. 5 mSv	(0.5 rem)
3. Equivalent dose limits for tissues and organs‡		
a. Lens of eye	7. 15 mSv	(1.5 rem)
b. Localized areas of the skin, hands, and feet	8. 50 mSv	(5 rem)
4. Remedial action for natural sources		
a. Effective dose (excluding radon)	9. >5 mSv	(>0.5 rem)
b. Exposure to radon and its decay products§	10. >0.007 Jhm^{-3}	(>2 WLM)
D. Education and training exposures (annual)‡		
1. Effective dose limit	11. 1 mSv	(0.1 rem)
2. Equivalent dose limit for tissues and organs		
a. Lens of eye	12. 15 mSv	(1.5 rem)
b. Localized areas of the skin, hands, and feet	13. 50 mSv	(5 rem)
E. Embryo-fetus exposures‡		
Equivalent dose limit		
a. Monthly	14. 0.5 mSv	(0.05 rem)
b. Entire gestation	15. 5.0 mSv	(0.5 rem)
F. Negligible individual dose (annual)‡	0.01 mSv	(0.001 rem)

*Excluding medical exposures.

†See Tables 4.2 and 5.1 in NCRP Report #116 for recommendations on radiation weighting factors and tissue weighting factors, respectively.

‡Sum of external and internal exposures, excluding doses from natural sources.

§WLM stands for working level month and refers to a cumulative exposure for a working month (170 hours). As applied to radon and its daughter products, 1 WLM represents the cumulative exposure experienced in a 170-hour period resulting from a radon concentration of 100 pCi/L. The occupational limit for miners is 4 WLM per year, which results in a dose equivalent of approximately 0.15 Sv (15 rem) per year.

Exercise 7—Short Answer

1. Exposure of the general public, patients, and radiation workers to ionizing radiation must be limited to minimize the risk of harmful biologic effects.

2. Medical imaging professionals must be familiar with previous, existing, and new guidelines because they share the responsibility for patient safety with radiation exposure and they also are subject to such exposure in the performance of their duties. By keeping themselves informed, they will be more conscious of good radiation safety practices.

3. Four major organizations that are responsible for evaluating the relationship between radiation equivalent dose (EqD) and induced biologic effects are the International Commission on Radiological Protection (ICRP); the National Council on Radiation Protection and Measurements (NCRP); the U.N. Scientific Committee on the Effects of Atomic Radiation (UNSCEAR); and the National Academy of Sciences/National Research Council Committee on the Biological Effects of Ionizing Radiation (NAS/NRC-BEIR).

4. Five U.S. regulatory agencies are responsible for enforcing radiation protection standards to safeguard the general public, patients, and occupationally exposed personnel: the Nuclear Regulatory Commission (NRC); states who have signed an NRC agreement; the Environmental Protection Agency (EPA); the Food and Drug Administration (FDA); and the Occupational Safety and Health Administration (OSHA).

5. The NRC mandates that a radiation safety committee (RSC) be established for a health care facility to assist in the development of radiation safety programs. This committee provides guidance for the program and facilitates its continuing operation.

6. The necessary training and experience for a radiation safety officer (RSO) are described in sections 10CFR35.50 and 10CFR35.900 of the Code of Federal Regulations. Three training pathways are specified: (1) certification by one of the professional boards approved by the NRC; (2) didactic and work experience as described in detail in the regulations; and (3) identification as an authorized user, authorized medical physicist, or authorized nuclear physicist on the license, with experience in the types of use for which the individual has RSO responsibility.

7. To define the designation *as low as reasonably achievable (ALARA),* health care facilities usually adopt investigation levels, defined as Level I and Level II. In the United States these levels traditionally are one tenth to three tenths the applicable regulatory limits.

8. Radiation protection has two explicit objectives: (1) to prevent any clinically important radiation-induced nonstochastic (deterministic) effect by adhering to dose limits beneath the threshold levels and (2) to limit the risk of stochastic responses to conservative levels as weighted against societal needs, values, benefits acquired, and economic considerations.

9. Occupational risk associated with radiation exposure may be equated with occupational risk in other industries generally considered reasonably safe (i.e., about 10^{-4} to 10^{-6} annually, meaning an excess cancer risk of one chance in 10,000 to one chance in 1 million per year). The risk generally is estimated to be a 2.5% chance of a fatal accident over an entire career.

10. The Consumer-Patient Radiation Health and Safety Act of 1981 carries no legal penalty for noncompliance, therefore several states simply have not responded with appropriate legislation.

11. When ionizing radiation damages reproductive cells, mutations may develop that could have deleterious consequences in subsequent generations. An example of this is effects on offspring caused by irradiation of reproductive cells (sperm and ova) before conception. This effect is called *mutagenesis.*

12. Two all-inclusive categories that encompass the radiation-induced responses of serious concern in radiation protection programs are nonstochastic (deterministic) effects and stochastic (probabilistic) effects.

13. The purpose of the Consumer-Patient Radiation Health and Safety Act of 1981 is to ensure that standard medical and dental radiologic procedures adhere to rigorous safety precautions and standards.

14. The EPA was established on December 2, 1970, to bring several agencies into one organization responsible for protecting the health of human beings and for safeguarding the natural environment.

15. Exposure linearity is defined as consistency in output radiation intensity at a selected KVp setting when changing from one milliamperage and time combination to another.

Exercise 8—Essay

The questions in this exercise are intended to allow students to express their knowledge and understanding of the subject matter covered in this chapter. Because the answers may vary, determination of an answer's acceptability is left to the discretion of the instructor.

Exercise 9—Calculation Problems

1. EqD = 10 mSv × Age (yr)
   EqD = 10 mSv × 54
   EqD = 540 mSv
2. EqD = Age in rem
   EqD = 54 rem
3. EqD = 10 mSv × Age (yr)
   EqD = 10 mSv × 46
   EqD = 460 mSv
4. EqD = Age in rem
   EqD = 46 rem
5. EqD = 10 mSv × Age (yr)
   EqD = 10 mSv × 33
   EqD = 330 mSv
6. EqD = Age in rem
   EqD = 33 rem
7. EqD = 10 mSv × Age (yr)
   EqD = 10 mSv × 25
   EqD = 250 mSv
8. EqD = Age in rem
   EqD = 25 rem
9. EqD = 10 mSv × Age (yr)
   EqD = 10 mSv × 18
   EqD = 180 mSv
10. EqD = Age in rem
    EqD = 18 rem

Post Test

1. In the medical industry, with reference to the radiation sciences, *risk* is the possibility of inducing a radiogenic cancer or genetic defect after irradiation.
2. national security
3. Occupational Safety and Health Administration (OSHA)
4. the radiation safety officer (RSO)
5. EqD = 10 mSv × Age (yr)
   EqD = 10 mSv × 39
   EqD = 390 mSv
6. EqD = Age in rem
   EqD = 39 rem
7. effective dose-limiting system
8. ALARA is the acronym for *as low as reasonably achievable.*
9. B
10. C
11. estimated
12. linear nonthreshold
13. occupational risk in other industries generally considered reasonably safe
14. The essential concept underlying radiation protection is that any organ in the human body is vulnerable to damage from exposure to ionizing radiation.
15. The NCRP now recommends an EqD limit of 5 mSv (0.5 rem) during the entire period of gestation.
16. 50 mSv (5 rem)
17. Accounting for tissue weighting factors is important because various tissues and organs do not have the same degree of sensitivity.
18. effective
19. *Radiation hormesis* is the hypothesis that a positive effect exists for certain populations that are continuously exposed to moderate levels of radiation.
20. Internal action limits are established by health care facilities to trigger an investigation to uncover the reasons for any unusual high exposures received by individual staff members.

Chapter 8

Exercise 1—Crossword Puzzle

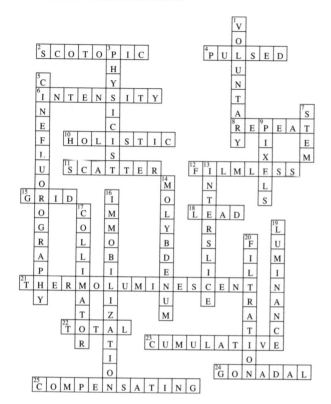

Exercise 2—Matching

1. N	6. O	11. U	16. A	21. V
2. I	7. Y	12. C	17. T	22. D
3. L	8. F	13. S	18. G	23. X
4. J	9. P	14. H	19. Q	24. B
5. K	10. E	15. W	20. M	25. R

Exercise 3—Multiple Choice

1. D	6. A	11. D	16. D	21. B
2. B	7. D	12. C	17. A	22. B
3. A	8. D	13. C	18. B	23. C
4. A	9. D	14. A	19. C	24. A
5. C	10. A	15. B	20. B	25. D

Exercise 4—True or False

1. T
2. F (Patients do need to be given the opportunity.)
3. F (These are x-ray beam limitation devices.)
4. T
5. F (inherent amounts to 0.5 mm aluminum equivalent)
6. T
7. F (They need to be selectively shielded.)
8. F (may be reduced by 90% to 95%)
9. T
10. T
11. F (higher kVp, lower mAs)
12. T
13. F (Radiation shielding requirements are decreased because of the reduction of x-radiation in the environment.)
14. F (The patient dose increases.)
15. F (It is not acceptable.)
16. F (The radiation dose to the breast of a young patient may be further reduced by performing the scoliosis examination with the x-ray beam entering the posterior surface of the patient's body instead of the anterior surface.)
17. T
18. T
19. T
20. F (the use of carbon fiber)
21. T
22. F (necessitate a decrease in peak kilovoltage by as much as 25%)
23. F (2-mm lead equivalent)
24. T
25. T

Exercise 5—Fill in the Blank

1. reduction, protective, minimize
2. limitation
3. respect
4. poor
5. decreases
6. female, male
7. reduces
8. symphysis pubis
9. wedge
10. electronic
11. same
12. distance
13. Standardized, high, lower
14. clinical interest
15. 0.2, (20)
16. 90, 95
17. shadow
18. minimal
19. density
20. workstations
21. unethical, unacceptable
22. dose reduction
23. dead-man
24. entrance, exit
25. pregnancy, menstrual period

Exercise 6—Labeling

A.

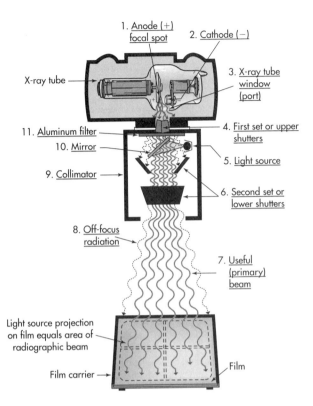

1. Anode (+) focal spot

2. Cathode (−)

X-ray tube

3. X-ray tube window (port)

11. Aluminum filter

10. Mirror

9. Collimator

4. First set or upper shutters

5. Light source

6. Second set or lower shutters

8. Off-focus radiation

7. Useful (primary) beam

Light source projection on film equals area of radiographic beam

Film carrier

Film

B.

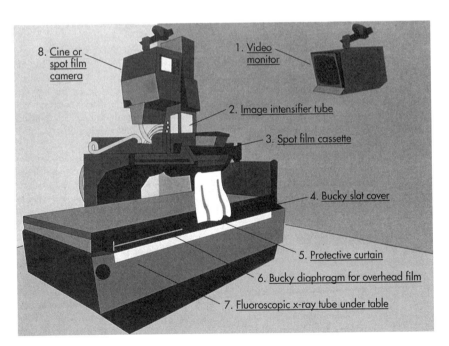

8. Cine or spot film camera

1. Video monitor

2. Image intensifier tube

3. Spot film cassette

4. Bucky slot cover

5. Protective curtain

6. Bucky diaphragm for overhead film

7. Fluoroscopic x-ray tube under table

From *Mosby's radiographic instructional series: radiobiology and radiation protection*, St Louis, 1999, Mosby.

C.

HVL Required by the Radiation Control for Health and Safety Act of 1968 and Detailed by the Bureau of Radiological Health* in 1980

Peak Kilovoltage	Minimum Required HVL in Millimeters of Aluminum
30	1. <u>0.3</u>
40	2. <u>0.4</u>
50	3. <u>1.2</u>
60	4. <u>1.3</u>
70	5. <u>1.5</u>
80	6. <u>2.3</u>
90	7. <u>2.5</u>
100	8. <u>2.7</u>
110	9. <u>3.0</u>
120	10. <u>3.2</u>

*The Bureau of Radiological Health changed its name to the Center for Devices and Radiological Health in 1982.

Exercise 7—Short Answer

1. During a radiographic procedure, radiographers can limit exposure of the patient to ionizing radiation by using appropriate radiation reduction techniques and protective devices that minimize radiation exposure. Patient exposure can be substantially reduced by using proper body and/or part immobilization, motion reduction techniques, appropriate beam limitation devices, adequate filtration of the x-ray beam, and gonadal or other specific area shielding. Selection of suitable technical exposure factors, in conjunction with either high-speed film-screen combinations or computer-generated digital images, correct radiographic film processing techniques, or appropriate digital image processing, as well as elimination of repeat radiographic exposures, also can help significantly limit patient exposure.

2. The first set of shutters in the collimator, the upper shutters, are mounted as close as possible to the x-ray tube window to reduce the amount of off-focus, or stem, radiation coming from the primary beam and exiting at various angles from the x-ray tube window. This radiation can never be completely eliminated because the metal shutters cannot be placed immediately beneath the actual focal spot of the x-ray tube; however, placing the upper shutters as close as possible to the tube window can reduce it significantly. This practice reduces patient exposure to off-focus radiation.

3. The four basic types of gonadal shielding devices that can be used during a radiologic procedure are flat contact shields, shadow shields, shaped contact shields, and clear lead shields.

4. Poorly processed radiographs offer inadequate diagnostic information, leading to repeat exposures and unnecessary patient radiation exposure.

5. Protective shielding is a structure or device made of certain materials (e.g., concrete, lead, or lead-impregnated material) that will adequately attenuate ionizing radiation.

6. For an air gap technique, the image receptor is placed 6 to 10 inches (15 to 25 cm) from the patient, and the x-ray tube is placed approximately 10 to 12 feet (2.7 to 3.6 m) from the image receptor. The scattered x-rays produced in the patient are disseminated in many directions at acute angles to the primary beam when the radiographic exposure is made. Because of this and the increased distance between the anatomy imaged and the image receptor, a higher percentage of the scattered x-rays are less likely to strike the image receptor. The air gap method results in an adequate grid-type scatter clean-up effect. In general, the air gap technique requires the selec-

tion of technical exposure factors comparable to those used with an 8:1 ratio grid. Therefore the patient dose is higher than that for a nongrid technique. The dose from an air gap technique is about the same as that for a midratio grid (8:1).

7. Inherent filtration includes the glass envelope encasing the x-ray tube, the insulating oil surrounding the tube, and the glass window in the x-ray tube housing.

8. Three reasons for high radiation exposure during interventional procedures performed by a physician who is not a radiologist are (1) the fluoroscopic tube may be operated for longer periods in continuous, rather than pulsed mode; (2) the protective curtain, or floating shields, on the stationary fluoroscopic equipment's image intensifier may not be used as a means of protection; and (3) cine frequently is used as a recording medium.

9. Four ways to specify the amount of radiation a patient receives from a diagnostic imaging procedure are entrance skin exposure (ESE), skin dose, gonadal dose, and bone marrow dose.

10. Direct patient shielding is not typically used in computed tomography (CT). Because of the rotational nature of the exposure, a shield is no more effective than the collimators already on the device. Because the beam is so tightly collimated to the slice thickness, exposure to the anatomy outside the field of view usually is caused only by internal scatter. Generally, with CT, anatomy does not appear in the primary x-ray beam unless it is part of the intended field of view.

11. Because filtration absorbs some of the photons in the radiographic beam, it decreases the overall intensity (amount, or quantity) of radiation.

12. Added filtration is located outside the glass window of the x-ray tube housing, above the collimator shutters.

13. Seven factors that must be considered in the selection of technical exposure factors are (1) the mass per unit volume of tissue of the area of clinical interest; (2) the effective atomic numbers and electron densities of the tissues involved; (3) the film-screen combination or other type of image receptor; (4) the source-to-image distance (SID); (5) the type and quantity of filtration used; (6) the type of x-ray generator used (single phase, three phase, or high frequency); and (7) the balance of radiographic density and contrast required.

14. Three benefits of a repeat analysis program are (1) the program increases awareness among staff and student radiographers of the need to produce optimal quality recorded images; (2) radiographers generally become more careful in producing images because they are aware that the images are reviewed; and (3) when the repeat analysis program identifies problems or concerns, in-service education programs covering these specific topics may be designed for imaging personnel.

15. Six x-ray procedures now considered nonessential are (1) a chest x-ray examination on scheduled admission to the hospital; (2) a chest x-ray examination as part of a preemployment physical; (3) a lumbar spine examination as part of a preemployment physical; (4) chest x-rays or other unjustified x-ray examinations as part of a routine health checkup; (5) a chest x-ray examination for mass screening for tuberculosis; and (6) a whole-body multislice spiral CT screening procedure.

16. Seven categories that may be established for discarded radiographs are (1) Too dark or too light because of inappropriate selection of technical exposure factors; (2) incorrect patient positioning; (3) incorrect centering of the radiographic beam; (4) patient motion during the radiographic exposure; (5) improper collimation of the radiographic beam; (6) presence of external foreign bodies; and (7) processing artifacts.

17. Eleven procedures involving extended fluoroscopic time are (1) percutaneous transluminal angioplasty, (2) radiofrequency cardiac catheter ablation, (3) vascular embolization, (4) stent and filter placement, (5) thrombolytic and fibrinolytic procedures, (6) percu-

taneous transhepatic cholangiography, (7) endoscopic retrograde cholangiopancreatography, (8) transjugular intrahepatic portosystemic shunt, (9) percutaneous nephrostomy, (10) biliary drainage, and (11) urinary or biliary stone removal.

18. The resettable cumulative timing device on fluoroscopic equipment times the x-ray beam-on time and sounds an audible alarm or temporarily interrupts the exposure after the fluoroscope has been activated for 5 minutes. It makes the radiologist aware of the length of time the patient receives exposure for each fluoroscopic examination.

19. For dose reduction purposes, whenever possible it is best to position the C-arm so that the x-ray tube is under the patient. Scatter radiation is less intense with the x-ray tube in this position. When the tube is positioned over the patient, scatter radiation becomes more intense, and the patient dose increases accordingly.

20. A small, relatively thin pack of thermoluminescent dosimeters (TLDs) is secured to the patient's skin in the middle of the clinical area of interest and exposed during a radiographic procedure. Because lithium fluoride (LiF), the sensing material in the TLD, responds similarly to human tissue when exposed to ionizing radiation, the surface dose can be accurately determined.

Exercise 8—Essay

The questions in this exercise are intended to allow students to express their knowledge and understanding of the subject matter covered in this chapter. Because the answers may vary, determination of an answer's acceptability is left to the discretion of the instructor.

Post Test

1. 10
2. F. B. Reynold stated the official position of the American College of Radiology at a press conference on October 20, 1976: "Abdominal radiological exams that have been requested after full consideration of the clinical status of a patient, including the possibility of pregnancy, need not be postponed or selectively scheduled."
3. double dose
4. Light-localizing variable-aperture rectangular collimator
5. The genetically significant dose (GSD) is the equivalent dose to the reproductive organs that, if received by every human being, would be expected to cause an identical gross genetic injury to the total population as does the sum of the actual doses received by exposed individual population members.
6. Use of a radiographic grid results in an increase in the patient dose.
7. effective
8. D
9. B
10. collimated
11. quantum mottle
12. interventional procedures
13. 50
14. The radiologist should use the practice of intermittent, or pulsed, fluoroscopy to reduce the overall length of exposure.
15. D
16. Both the alignment and the length and width dimensions of the radiographic beam must correspond to within 2% of the source-to-image distance (SID).
17. three
18. The symphysis pubis can be used to guide shield placement over the testes.
19. D
20. projections

Chapter 9

Exercise 1—Crossword Puzzle

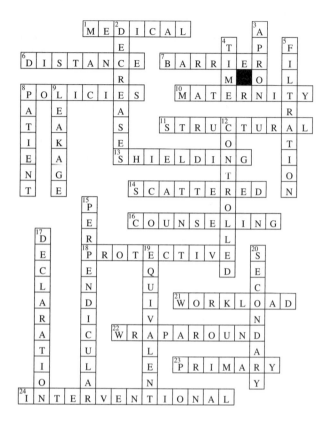

Exercise 2—Matching

1. C	6. U	11. J	16. V	21. E
2. P	7. I	12. T	17. B	22. Y
3. F	8. O	13. A	18. N	23. H
4. S	9. Q	14. G	19. X	24. D
5. K	10. L	15. R	20. M	25. W

Exercise 3—Multiple Choice

1. A	6. D	11. C	16. D	21. D
2. D	7. D	12. D	17. C	22. D
3. D	8. D	13. C	18. D	23. A
4. D	9. A	14. B	19. C	24. A
5. B	10. B	15. D	20. D	25. D

Exercise 4—True or False

1. T
2. F (Personal medical and natural background radiation exposure are not included.)
3. T
4. T
5. F (inversely proportional)
6. F (0.5-mm lead equivalency)
7. F (0.25-mm thickness of lead)
8. T
9. F (Bucky slot shielding device)
10. T
11. F (limits the methods that can be used to achieve protection)
12. T
13. F (A radiographer should never stand in the useful beam to restrain a patient during a radiographic exposure.)
14. T
15. T
16. F (primarily benefits the patient)
17. F (as a consequence of the Compton scattering process)
18. T
19. T
20. F (Diagnostic imaging department staff members who are pregnant should be able to continue performing their duties without interruption of employment if they follow radiation safety practices.)
21. F (directly proportional)
22. T
23. T
24. T
25. F (During fluoroscopic examinations, the radiographer should always wear a protective apron.)

Exercise 5—Fill in the Blank

1. equivalent
2. Scattered
3. decrease, reduction
4. safety
5. increased
6. Shortening
7. distance
8. shielding
9. aprons, gloves, thyroid shields
10. housing, high-tension
11. Compton scatter, Compton scatter
12. 0.5 (0.05), 5 (0.5)
13. 0.5-mm, 1-mm
14. time, distance, shielding
15. four, four
16. perpendicular
17. $^{1}/_{16}$ inch, 7 (2.1)
18. $^{1}/_{32}$ inch
19. 0.5-mm
20. scattered, patient, assistance
21. 0.25 mm
22. radiologist, control-booth barrier
23. wraparound
24. right angles (90), least
25. routine

Exercise 6—Labeling

A.

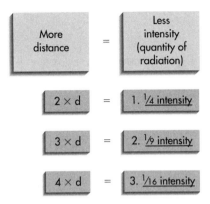

More distance	=	Less intensity (quantity of radiation)
$2 \times d$	=	1. ¼ intensity
$3 \times d$	=	2. ⅑ intensity
$4 \times d$	=	3. 1/16 intensity

B.

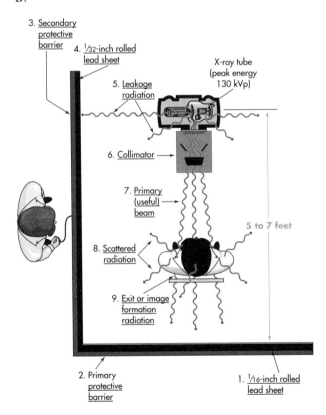

3. Secondary protective barrier
4. 1/32-inch rolled lead sheet
X-ray tube (peak energy 130 kVp)
5. Leakage radiation
6. Collimator
7. Primary (useful) beam
5 to 7 feet
8. Scattered radiation
9. Exit or image formation radiation
2. Primary protective barrier
1. 1/16-inch rolled lead sheet

C.

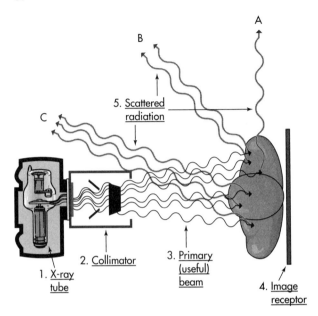

A
B
C
5. Scattered radiation
1. X-ray tube
2. Collimator
3. Primary (useful) beam
4. Image receptor

Exercise 7—Short Answer

1. The occupational risk for monitored diagnostic imaging personnel can be compared with the occupational risk for people employed in other industries generally considered to be reasonably safe, such as government and trade. These jobs have a risk of fatal accidents generally estimated to be about $1 \times 10^{-4} \ y^{-1}$.

2. Lead aprons are designed to provide protection from secondary (leakage and scatter) radiation.

3. When high-speed imaging receptor systems are used, a smaller radiographic exposure (less milliamperage) is required, therefore fewer x-ray photons are available to produce Compton scatter. The reduction in Compton scatter reduces occupational exposure of the radiographer.

4. Most health care facilities have policies for protecting pregnant personnel from radiation. Under these policies an imaging professional who becomes pregnant first informs her supervisor. After this voluntary "declaration" has been made, the health care facility officially recognizes the pregnancy. The facility, through its radiation safety officer, provides essential counseling and furnishes an appropriate additional monitor.

5. The three basic principles of radiation protection are time, distance, and shielding.

6. A qualified medical physicist will determine the exact requirements for protective structural shielding for a particular imaging facility.

7. Protective aprons, gloves, and thyroid shields are made of lead-impregnated vinyl.

8. Diagnostic imaging personnel can substantially reduce scatter radiation to the lens of the eyes by wearing protective eyeglasses with optically clear lenses that have a minimal lead equivalent protection of 0.35 mm. Side shields on the glasses are also available for procedures that require turning of the head. A wraparound frame containing optically clear lenses with a 0.5-mm lead equivalency is also available.

9. A lead-lined, metal, diagnostic-type protective tube housing protects both the radiographer and the patient from off-focus, or leakage, radiation by restricting the emission of x-rays to the area of the useful, or primary, beam.

181

10. Remote control fluoroscopic systems provide the best radiation protection for imaging personnel. These systems allow the radiologist and assisting radiographer to remain outside the fluoroscopy room at a control console behind a protective barrier until needed. This increases imaging personnel safety because distance is used as a means of increased protection. With remote equipment the radiologist and assisting radiographer can view the patient directly through clear protective shielding and enter the x-ray room only when absolutely necessary to provide essential patient care or perform procedural functions.

11. Positioning of a C-arm fluoroscope with the x-ray tube over the table and the image intensifier underneath the table results in higher patient exposure and increased scatter radiation. As scatter increases, radiation exposure of all personnel in the immediate vicinity of the C-arm also increases. From the perspective of increased radiation safety, therefore, it is best to reverse the C-arm to place the x-ray tube under the table and the image intensifier over the table.

12. Exposure of personnel is caused by scatter radiation from the patient. During operating room procedures in which cross-table exposures are made with a mobile C-arm fluoroscope, an understanding of the patterns of x-ray scatter is particularly useful. The exposure rate caused by scatter near the entrance surface of the patient (the x-ray tube side) exceeds the exposure rate caused by scatter near the exit surface of the patient (the image intensifier side). The difference in the amount of scatter, typically a factor of two or three, is caused by the higher radiation intensity at the entrance surface of the patient. Thus the location of the lower potential scatter dose is on the side of the patient away from the x-ray tube (i.e., the image intensifier side).

13. The radiologist or other interventional physician can reduce radiation exposure during a high-level-control interventional procedure by shortening the duration of the procedure, thereby reducing fluoroscopic beam-on time; taking fewer digital and cineradiographic images; reducing the use of continuous mode (as opposed to pulsed mode) of operation; keeping the protective curtain, if present, on the image intensifier or scatter shield in place during a procedure; and by regularly using the last-image-hold feature to view the most recent fluoroscopic images. These safety practices substantially reduce exposure to all participating personnel and also to the patient.

14. Because the hands and forearms of physicians performing interventional procedures can be subjected to large radiation exposures if the safety protocol is not followed carefully (which sometimes may not be possible), monitoring of the extremities is crucial. Physicians need to be aware of the recommended dose limits that have been established for the extremities. The National Council of Radiation Protection and Measurements (NCRP) currently recommends an annual equivalent dose limit to localized areas of the skin and hands of 500 mSv (50 rem). To avoid remotely approaching this limit and consequently increasing the possibility of adverse effects, any physician whose hands often need to be close to the fluoroscopic beam should wear protective gloves whenever possible.

15. Eight radiation-absorbent barrier design considerations are (1) the mean energy of the x-ray beam that will strike the barrier; (2) whether the barrier is a primary or secondary one; (3) the distance from the x-ray source to a position of occupancy 1 foot (30 cm) from the barrier; (4) the workload of the unit; (5) the use factor of the unit; (6) the occupancy factor behind the barrier; (7) the intrinsic shielding (e.g., tube housing attenuation of the x-ray unit); and (8) whether the area beyond the barrier is controlled or uncontrolled.

Exercise 8—Essay

The questions in this exercise are intended to allow students to express their knowledge and understanding of the subject matter covered in this chapter. Because the answers may vary, determination of an answer's acceptability is left to the discretion of the instructor.

Exercise 9—Calculation Problems

1.
$$\frac{I_1}{I_2} = \frac{(d_2)^2}{(d_1)^2}$$
$$\frac{9}{I_2} = \frac{(6)^2}{(3)^2}$$
$$\frac{9}{I_2} = \frac{36}{9} \text{ (cross-multiply)}$$
$$36I_2 = 81$$
$$I_2 = 2.25 \text{ mR/hr}$$

2.
$$\frac{I_1}{I_2} = \frac{(d_2)^2}{(d_1)^2}$$
$$\frac{5}{I_2} = \frac{(4)^2}{(2)^2}$$
$$\frac{5}{I_2} = \frac{16}{4} \text{ (cross-multiply)}$$
$$16I_2 = 20$$
$$I_2 = 1.25 \text{ mR/hr}$$

3.
$$\frac{I_1}{I_2} = \frac{(d_2)^2}{(d_1)^2}$$
$$\frac{4}{I_2} = \frac{(10)^2}{(5)^2}$$
$$\frac{4}{I_2} = \frac{100}{25} \text{ (cross-multiply)}$$
$$100I_2 = 100$$
$$I_2 = 1 \text{ mR/hr}$$

4.
$$\frac{I_1}{I_2} = \frac{(d_2)^2}{(d_1)^2}$$
$$\frac{7}{I_2} = \frac{(2)^2}{(1)^2}$$
$$\frac{7}{I_2} = \frac{4}{1} \text{ (cross-multiply)}$$
$$4I_2 = 7$$
$$I_2 = 1.75 \text{ mR/hr}$$

5.
$$\frac{I_1}{I_2} = \frac{(d_2)^2}{(d_1)^2}$$
$$\frac{6}{I_2} = \frac{(12)^2}{(6)^2}$$
$$\frac{6}{I_2} = \frac{144}{36} \text{ (cross-multiply)}$$
$$144I_2 = 216$$
$$I_2 = 1.5 \text{ mR/hr}$$

6.
$$\frac{I_1}{I_2} = \frac{(d_2)^2}{(d_1)^2}$$
$$\frac{6}{I_2} = \frac{(6)^2}{(2)^2}$$
$$\frac{6}{I_2} = \frac{36}{24} \text{ (cross-multiply)}$$
$$36I_2 = 24$$
$$I_2 = 0.666 \text{ mR/hr}$$

7. $(10/5)^2$ $10 \div 5 = 2$ $2 \times 2 = 4$
8. $(12/4)^2$ $12 \div 4 = 3$ $3 \times 3 = 9$
9. $(4/1)^2$ $4 \div 1 = 4$ $4 \times 4 = 16$
10. $(8/2)^2$ $8 \div 2 = 4$ $4 \times 4 = 16$

Post Test

1. Distance
2. declaration
3. The genetically significant dose (GSD) is the equivalent dose to the reproductive organs that, if received by every human being, would be expected to cause an identical gross genetic injury to the total population as does the sum of the actual doses received by exposed individual population members.
4. Scattered radiation
5. gonadal
6. The intensity of radiation is inversely proportional to the square of the distance from the source.
7. restrain
8. Time, distance and shielding
9. D
10. B
11. B
12. records
13. thickness
14. scattered

15.
$$\frac{I_1}{I_2} = \frac{(d_2)^2}{(d_1)^2}$$

$$\frac{10}{I_2} = \frac{(6)^2}{(3)^2}$$

$$\frac{10}{I_2} = \frac{36}{9} \text{ (cross-multiply)}$$

$$36I_2 = 90$$
$$I_2 = 2.5 \text{ mR/hr}$$

16. Secondary protective barrier
17. patient
18. 500 mSv (50 rem)
19. radiographer
20. 0.5, (0.05)

Chapter 10

Exercise 1—Crossword Puzzle

Across: 3. PERSONNEL; 7. LIGHTWEIGHT; 8. ELECTROMETER; 11. THERMOLUMINESCENT; 12. LUMINESCENCE; 13. TWO; 14. COPPER; 16. CALIBRATION; 19. IMMEDIATE; 20. FUZZY; 21. GESTATION; 22. EXTREMITY; 23. DARKEN

Exercise 2—Matching

1. K	6. N	11. Y	16. Q	21. J
2. M	7. B	12. W	17. D	22. S
3. L	8. O	13. R	18. G	23. X
4. C	9. A	14. P	19. E	24. V
5. H	10. I	15. U	20. F	25. T

Exercise 3—Multiple Choice

1. D	6. B	11. A	16. A	21. A
2. B	7. C	12. D	17. C	22. C
3. A	8. C	13. D	18. D	23. A
4. C	9. B	14. D	19. A	24. D
5. C	10. A	15. A	20. A	25. B

Exercise 4—True or False

1. F (They do not protect the wearer from ionizing radiation.)
2. T
3. T
4. F (It is a factor; personnel dosimeters selected for use must be cost-effective.)
5. F (should be made of plastic of a low atomic number)
6. F (Exposure time is too short to allow the meter to respond.)
7. T
8. T
9. F (not equally sensitive in the detection of ionizing radiation)
10. T
11. F (usually for 1 month)
12. T
13. T
14. F (made out of aluminum, copper, and tin)
15. T
16. T
17. F (An optically stimulated luminescence dosimeter [OSL] can be worn up to 1 year; it commonly is worn for 2 months.)
18. T
19. T
20. F (A thermoluminescent dosimeter [TLD] can be read only once because the reading destroys the stored information.)
21. T
22. T
23. T
24. T
25. T

Exercise 5—Fill in the Blank

1. thyroid, eyes
2. detect, record
3. ionization, optically stimulated, thermoluminescent
4. inexpensive
5. sharply defined
6. radiation-free
7. equivalent
8. trigger
9. charged, zero
10. common
11. sensitive
12. lost, contamination
13. calibrate
14. occupational
15. 1, 0.5 (50)
16. dosimeter
17. deep, shallow
18. reused, cost-effective
19. Control
20. body
21. densitometer
22. worn
23. legal
24. 5, 40
25. plastic

183

Exercise 6—Labeling

A.

Personnel Monitoring Devices Currently Available

1. Film badge
2. Extremity dosimeter (TLD ring badge)
3. Optically stimulated luminescence dosimeter (OSL)
4. Pocket ionization chamber (pocket dosimeter)
5. Thermoluminescent dosimeter (TLD)

Exercise 7—Short Answer

1. Personnel dosimeters provide an indication of the working habits and working conditions of diagnostic imaging personnel.
2. Four types of personnel dosimeters are used to measure individual exposure of the body to ionizing radiation: film badges, OSL dosimeters, pocket ionization chambers, and TLDs.
3. An extremity dosimeter measures the approximate equivalent dose to the hands of the wearer of the dosimeter.
4. The badge cover of an extremity monitor contains information such as the account number, participant's name and number, wear date, indication of hand (right or left), size, and reference number of the TLD ring dosimeter. All of this is laser etched to ensure permanent identification.
5. Optical density is the intensity of light transmitted through a given area of the medical imaging film.
6. Three radiation survey instruments used for area monitoring are the ionization chamber–type survey meter (cutie pie), the proportional counter, and the Geiger-Müller (G-M) detector.
7. Proportional counters are generally used in a laboratory to detect alpha and beta radiation and small amounts of other types of low-level radioactive contamination.
8. Some disadvantages of the TLD are (1) the initial high cost; (2) it can be read only once because the readout process destroys the stored information; and (3) calibrated dosimeters must be used with TLDs.
9. The OSL dosimeter contains an aluminum oxide (Al_2O_3) detector (thin layer).
10. Radiation dosimetry film is sensitive to doses ranging from as low as 0.1 mSv (10 mrem) to as high as 5000 mSv (500 rem).
11. Exposure monitoring of personnel is required whenever radiation workers are likely to risk receiving 10% or more of the annual occupational effective dose limit of 50 mSv (5 rem) in any single year.
12. When a protective lead apron is used during fluoroscopy or special procedures, the personnel dosimeter should be worn outside the apron at collar level on the anterior surface of the body because the unprotected head, neck, and lenses of the eye receive 10 to 20 times more exposure than the protected body trunk. When the personnel dosimeter is located at collar level, it also provides a reading of the approximate equivalent dose to the thyroid gland and eyes of the occupationally exposed person.
13. Occupational exposure values found on a record of radiation exposure represent the average annual effective dose (EfD) to the whole body.
14. When the letter "M" appears under the current monitoring period or in the cumulative columns of a personnel monitoring report, it signifies that an equivalent dose below the minimum measurable radiation quantity was recorded during that time.
15. When changing employment, a radiation worker must convey the data pertinent to the accumulated permanent equivalent dose to the new employer so that this information can be kept on file.

Exercise 8—Essay

The questions in this exercise are intended to allow students to express their knowledge and understanding of the subject matter covered in this chapter. Because the answers may vary, determination of an answer's acceptability is left to the discretion of the instructor.

Post Test

1. effective
2. An OSL dosimeter is a device for monitoring exposure that contains an aluminum oxide detector. When the dosimeter is read out, optically stimulated luminosity occurs when the dosimeter is struck by laser light at selected frequencies. When such laser light is incident on the sensing material, it becomes luminescent in proportion to the amount of radiation exposure received.
3. The working habits and conditions of diagnostic imaging personnel can be assessed over a designated period of time through the use of the personnel dosimeter.
4. results
5. at collar level
6. A
7. D
8. In a health care facility, a radiographer's deep, eye, and shallow occupational exposure as measured by an exposed monitor may be found on the personnel monitoring report.
9. A G-M detector
10. Zero (0)
11. abdomen
12. the data pertinent to the accumulated permanent equivalent dose so that it may be placed on file with the new employer
13. measure
14. employment
15. Radiation workers are required to wear personnel monitoring devices whenever they are likely to risk receiving 10% or more of the annual EfD limit.
16. primary
17. the radiation safety officer (RSO)
18. two
19. Ionization chambers
20. pregnant

Chapter 11

Exercise 1—Crossword Puzzle
(*See following page*)

Exercise 2—Matching

1. S	6. T	11. A	16. F	21. R
2. V	7. H	12. E	17. C	22. Q
3. K	8. O	13. Y	18. X	23. G
4. J	9. N	14. L	19. P	24. I
5. M	10. W	15. D	20. U	25. B

Exercise 3—Multiple Choice

1. C	6. D	11. C	16. D	21. C
2. C	7. A	12. B	17. B	22. C
3. D	8. C	13. D	18. C	23. C
4. C	9. B	14. B	19. D	24. D
5. C	10. A	15. C	20. B	25. C

Exercise 4—True or False

1. F (unstable)
2. T
3. T
4. F (unstable atom)
5. F (9 neutrons)
6. F (It is of concern to the general population.)

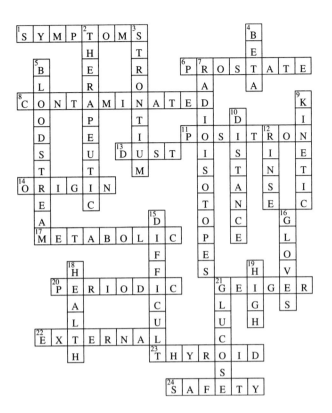

15. F (Geiger counters)
16. F (Radiation therapy uses ionizing radiation for the treatment of disease, namely, cancer.)
17. T
18. F (A positron is a form of antimatter.)
19. T
20. T
21. F (These 511 keV photons cannot be shielded by an ordinary lead apron.)
22. T
23. T
24. T
25. T

Exercise 5—Fill in the Blank

1. 90, adjacent
2. metastases
3. 6, nucleus
4. Positron
5. prep
6. radiation
7. dirty bomb
8. radiosensitive
9. beta
10. electron capture
11. patient
12. unstable
13. annihilation
14. metabolic
15. Geiger
16. vary
17. plastic container
18. pregnant, 6
19. calcium
20. residual, sparing
21. isolated, minimize
22. radiotracer
23. 9
24. full
25. Monitoring

7. T
8. T
9. F (They are useful.)
10. F (short-lived radioisotopes)
11. F (No, technetium-99m is.)
12. T
13. T
14. T

Exercise 6—Labeling

A.

Dose-Effect Relation After Acute Whole-Body Radiation from Gamma Rays or X-Rays*

Whole-Body Absorbed Dose	Effect
0.05 Gy	No symptoms
1. 0.15 Gy	No symptoms, but possible chromosomal aberrations in cultured peripheral-blood lymphocytes
2. 0.5 Gy	No symptoms (minor decreases in white-cell and platelet counts in a few persons)
3. 1 Gy	Nausea and vomiting in approximately 10 percent of patients within 48 hours after exposure
4. 2 Gy	Nausea and vomiting in approximately 50% of persons within 24 hr, with marked decreases in white-cell and platelet counts
5. 4 Gy	Nausea and vomiting in 90% of persons within 12 hr, and diarrhea in 10% within 8 hr; 50% mortality in the absence of medical treatment
6. 6 Gy	100% mortality within 30 days due to bone marrow failure in the absence of medical treatment
7. 10 Gy	Approximate dose that is survivable with the best medical therapy available
8. >10–30 Gy	Nausea and vomiting in all persons in less than 5 min; severe gastrointestinal damage; death likely in 2 to 3 wk in the absence of treatment
9. >30 Gy	Cardiovascular collapse and central nervous system damage, with death in 24 to 72 hr

*Gusev I, Guskova AK, Mettler FA Jr, editors: *Medical management of radiation accidents*, ed 2, Boca Raton, Fla., 2001, CRC Press.

185

Exercise 7—Short Answer

1. Therapeutic isotopes may be characterized by relatively long half-lives, which are measured in terms of multiple days or multiple years and (except for a few) quite high energy radiation. The radiation may be in the form of gamma rays or fast electrons (beta radiation).

2. Electron capture occurs when an inner shell electron is captured by one of the nuclear protons and the two combine, producing a neutron and thereby creating a different element.

3. The process of beta decay occurs when a nucleus relieves an instability through conversion of a neutron into a proton, and an electron, and a neutrino, with the emission of the electron and the neutrino.

4. Diagnostic techniques in nuclear medicine typically make use of short-lived radioisotopes as radioactive tracers. These radionuclides are attached to biologically active substances or chemicals, forming radioactive compounds that predominantly diffuse into certain regions or organs where particular physiologic processes require assessment.

5. Positron emission tomography (PET) is an important imaging modality because it allows examination of metabolic processes in the body. This is particularly important with regard to the proliferation of cancer cells.

6. Fluorodeoxyglucose (FDG) is a radioactive tracer that is very similar in chemical behavior to ordinary glucose and therefore is taken up or metabolized by cancerous cells; it also reveals the locations of these cells through its positron emission decay and subsequent generation of oppositely traveling annihilation photons. These annihilation event sites are localizable through the PET scanner's ring of coincidence detectors.

7. Combining a PET scanner and a computed tomography (CT) scanner in a tandem configuration to form a single imaging device has two advantages: the combination imager not only can detect abnormally high regions of glucose metabolism, yielding evidence of the spread of cancer or of metastasis to other body areas, but it at the same time can provide detailed information about the location and size of these lesions.

8. With the attack on the World Trade Center on September 11, 2001, the possible use of other terrorist weapons, such as radiation, became a public health concern.

9. The Environmental Protection Agency (EPA) sets limits for radioactive contamination that assume that a 1 in 10,000 risk of causing a fatal cancer resulting is unacceptable. This type of regulation requires hospitals, educational facilities, and industries to control accidental exposures so that the health of the population cannot be measurably affected. It also assumes that many other carcinogens are present and that all are regulated to a similarly low level.

10. Personnel should wear gowns, masks, and gloves when working with a patient who has surface radioactive contamination.

11. The health care facility's radiation safety officer.

12. Normal badge limits do not apply during a radiation emergency.

13. Medical management during the first 48 hours involves simply treating the symptoms (e.g., nausea and vomiting) and trying to prevent dehydration.

14. Annihilation radiation is radiation in the form of two oppositely moving, 511 keV photons generated as the result of mutual annihilation of matter and antimatter (i.e., an electron and a positron).

15. A radioactive dispersal device, or dirty bomb, is a radioactive source mixed with conventional explosives. When such a device explodes, it spreads radioactive material through a specific area, causing contamination and panic.

Exercise 8—Essay

The questions in this exercise are intended to allow students to express their knowledge and understanding of the subject matter covered in this chapter. Because the answers may vary, determination of an answer's acceptability is left to the discretion of the instructor.

Post Test

1. EPA
2. A radioactive dispersal device, or dirty bomb, is a radioactive source mixed with conventional explosives. When it explodes, this device spreads radioactive material through a specific area, causing contamination and panic.
3. Therapeutic radioisotopes are characterized by their relatively long half-lives.
4. B
5. neutrons
6. Rapidly
7. A neutrino is a particle that has negligible mass and no charge but carries away any excess energy from the nucleus of the atom.
8. After a dirty bomb explodes, externally contaminated individuals can be decontaminated by removing contaminated clothing and immersion in a shower.
9. Annihilation radiation
10. 2 (200)
11. FDG
12. short-lived
13. 250 mSv (25 rem)
14. Electron capture is a process in which an inner shell electron is captured by one of the nuclear protons and the two combine to produce a neutron, creating a different element.
15. Positron emitters result in the production of high-energy radiation.
16. Geiger-Müller (GM) detector (Geiger counter)
17. Technetium-99m
18. radiation emergency plan and trained personnel
19. high energy
20. Beta